Histological Typing of Cancer and Precancer of the Oral Mucosa

Springer
Berlin
Heidelberg
New York
Barcelona
Budapest
Hong Kong
London
Milan
Paris
Santa Clara
Singapore
Tokyo

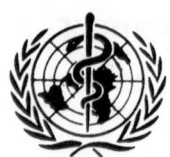 World Health Organization

The series *International Histological Classification of Tumours* consists of the following volumes. Each of these volumes – apart from volumes 1 and 2, which have already been revised – will appear in a revised edition within the next few years. Volumes of the current editions can be ordered through WHO, Distribution and Sales, Avenue Appia, CH-1211 Geneva 27.

1. Histological typing of lung tumours (1967, second edition 1981)
2. Histological typing of breast tumours (1968, second edition 1981)
4. Histological typing of oral and oropharyngeal tumours (1971)
8. Cytology of the female genital tract (1973)
9. Histological typing of ovarian tumours (1973)
10. Histological typing of urinary bladder tumours (1973)
14. Histological and cytological typing of neoplastic diseases of haematopoietic and lymphoid tissues (1976)
16. Histological typing of testis tumours (1977)
17. Cytology of non-gynaecological sites (1977)
22. Histological typing of prostate tumours (1980)
23. Histological typing of endocrine tumours (1980)
24. Histological typing of tumours of the eye and its adnexa (1980)
25. Histological typing of kidney tumours (1981)

A coded compendium of the International Histological Classification of Tumours (1978).

The following volumes have already appeared in a revised second edition with Springer-Verlag:
Histological Typing of Thyroid Tumours. Hedinger/Williams/Sobin (1988)
Histological Typing of Intestinal Tumours. Jass/Sobin (1989)
Histological Typing of Oesophageal and Gastric Tumours. Watanabe/Jass/Sobin (1990)
Histological Typing of Tumours of the Gallbladder and Extrahepatic Bile Ducts. Albores-Saavedra/Henson/Sobin (1990)
Histological Typing of Tumours of the Upper Respiratory Tract and Ear. Shanmugaratnam/Sobin (1981)
Histological Typing of Salivary Gland Tumours. Seifert (1991)
Histological Typing of Odontogenic Tumours. Kramer/Pindborg/Shear (1992)
Histological Typing of Tumours of the Central Nervous System. Kleihues/Burger/Scheithauer (1993)
Histological Typing of Bone Tumours. Schajowicz (1993)
Histological Typing of Soft Tissue Tumours. Weiss (1994)
Histological Typing of Female Genital Tract Tumours. Scully et al. (1994)
Histological Typing of Tumours of the Liver. Ishak et al. (1994)
Histological Typing of Tumours of the Exocrine Pancreas. Klöppel/Solcia/Longnecker/Capella/Sobin (1996)
Histological Typing of Skin Tumours. Heenan/Elder/Sobin (1996)
Histological Typing of Cancer and Precancer of the Oral Mucosa. Pindborg/Reichart/Smith/van der Waal (1997)

Histological Typing of Cancer and Precancer of the Oral Mucosa

J. J. Pindborg, P. A. Reichart,
C. J. Smith, and I. van der Waal

In Collaboration with L. H. Sobin
and Pathologists in 9 Countries

Second Edition

With 80 Colour Figures and 13 Drawings

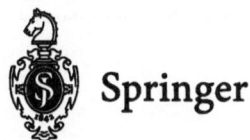 Springer

Dr. J. J. Pindborg †
Department of Oral Pathology, University of Copenhagen, Denmark

Dr. P. A. Reichart
Department of Oral Surgery and Oral Radiology,
Humboldt University of Berlin, Medical Faculty, Charité, Berlin, Germany

Dr. C. J. Smith
Department of Oral Pathology, University of Sheffield, England

Dr. I. van der Waal
Department of Oral Surgery and Oral Pathology,
Academic Hospital, Free University/ACTA, Amsterdam, The Netherlands

First edition published by WHO in 1971 in the International Histological Classification
of Tumours series

ISBN-13:978-3-540-61848-5

CIP Data applied for

Die Deutsche Bibliothek – CIP-Einheitsaufnahme
International histological classification of tumours / World Health Organization. – Berlin ; Heidel-
berg; New York ; London ; Paris ; Tokyo ; Hong Kong ; Barcelona ; Budapest : Springer.
NE: World Health Organization
Histological typing of cancer and precancer of the oral mucosa. – 2. ed. – 1997
Histological typing of cancer and precancer of the oral mucosa / [World Health Organization].
J. J. Pindborg . . . In collab. with L. H. Sobin and pathologists in 9 countries. – 2. ed. – Berlin ; Heidel-
berg ; New York ; Barcelona ; Budapest ; Hong Kong ; London ; Milan ; Paris ; Santa Clara ; Singa-
pore ; Tokyo : Springer, 1997
(International histological classification of tumours)
ISBN-13:978-3-540-61848-5   e-ISBN-13:978-3-642-60592-5
DOI:10.1007/978-3-642-60592-5

NE: Pindborg, Jens J.; World Health Organization

SPIN: 10552326   81/3135 – 5 4 3 2 1 0 – Printed on acid-free paper

Reviewers

Altini, M., Dr.
Department of Oral Pathology, University of The Witwaters-
rand, Johannesburg, South Africa

Anneroth, G., Dr.
Department of Oral Pathology, University of Umeå, Sweden

Bhonsle, R. B., Dr.
Oral Cancer Research Unit, Tata Institute of Fundamental
Research, Kerala, India

Bouquot, J. E., Dr.
The Maxillofacial Center, Morgantown, West Virginia, USA

Delgado, W., Dr.
Department of Oral Medicine, Oral Surgery and Oral Pathology, Universidad Peruana Cayetano Heredia, Lima, Peru

Ellis, G. L., Dr.
Department of Oral Pathology, Armed Forces Institute of
Pathology, Washington DC, USA

Kameyama, Y., Dr.
Department of Oral Pathology, Aichigakuin University, Nagoya,
Japan

Löning, Th., Dr.
Department of Gynecological Histopathology and Electron-
microscopy, University of Hamburg, Germany

Lucas-Tomas, M., Dr.
Department of Oral Medicine, Universidad Complutense de
Madrid, Spain

Murti, P. R., Dr.
Oral Cancer Research Unit, Tata Institute of Fundamental
Research, Kerala, India

Shanmugaratnam, K., Dr.
Department of Pathology, National University of Singapore,
Republic of Singapore

Sobin, L., Dr.
Division of Gastrointestinal Pathology, Armed Forces Institute
of Pathology, Washington DC, USA. (WHO Collaborating
Centre for the International Histological Classification of
Tumours)

General Preface to the Series

Among the prerequisites for comparative studies of cancer are international agreement on histological criteria for the definition and classification of cancer types and a standardized nomenclature. An internationally agreed classification of tumours, acceptable alike to physicians, surgeons, radiologists, pathologists and statisticians, would enable cancer workers in all parts of the world to compare their findings and would facilitate collaboration among them.

In a report published in 1952[1], a subcommittee of the World Health Organization (WHO) Expert Committee on Health Statistics discussed the general principles that should govern the statistical classification of tumours and agreed that, to ensure the necessary flexibility and ease of coding, three separate classifications were needed according to (1) anatomical site, (2) histological type, and (3) degree of malignancy. A classification according to anatomical site is available in the International Classification of Diseases[2].

In 1956, the WHO Executive Board passed a resolution[3] requesting the Director-General to explore the possibility that WHO might organize centres in various parts of the world and arrange for the collection of human tissues and their histological classification. The main purpose of such centres would be to develop histological definitions of cancer types and to facilitate the wide adoption of a uniform nomenclature. The resolution was endorsed by the Tenth World Health Assembly in May 1957[4].

---

[1] WHO (1952) WHO Technical Report Series, no. 53. WHO, Geneva, p 45
[2] WHO (1977) Manual of the international statistical classification of diseases, injuries, and causes of death, 1975 version. WHO, Geneva
[3] WHO (1956) WHO Official Records, no. 68, p 14 (resolution EB 17.R40)
[4] WHO (1957) WHO Official Records, no. 79, p 467 (resolution WHA 10.18)

Since 1958, WHO has established a number of centres concerned with this subject. The result of this endeavour has been the International Histological Classification of Tumours, a multi-volumed series whose first edition was published between 1967 and 1981. The present revised second edition aims to update the classification, reflecting progress in diagnosis and the relevance of tumour types to clinical and epidemiological features.

Preface to Histological Typing of Cancer and Precancer of the Oral Mucosa Second Edition

The publication of *Histological Typing of Oral and Oropharyngeal Tumours*[1] was the result of a collaborative effort organized by WHO and carried out by the International Reference/Collaborating Centre for the Histological Definition and Classification of Oral and Oropharyngeal Tumours at the Department of Pathology, Sarojini Naidu Medical College, Agra, India. The Centre was established in 1963 and the classification was published in 1971.

In 1967, WHO established a group to characterize and define the lesions that should be considered in a study of oral precancer and to determine, if possible, their relative risk of becoming malignant. This group published in 1978 an outline of the types of lesions under consideration and of some of their basic histopathological features.[2]

In order to keep the classification up to date and to meet the desire of WHO to merge the activities related to oral cancer and to oral precancer, a new international panel of consultants was established, listed on page IV, and were asked to prepare a draft text. After further preparatory work and discussion, a revised draft was sent to the reviewers listed on pages V–VI. Their comments were taken into account in the preparation of the final text. The authors express their sincere appreciation of the help so willingly given by the reviewers.

There were a few tumour types and conditions on which divergent views were expressed on the classification, terminology

---

[1] Wahi PN, Cohen B, Luthra U, Torloni H (1971) Histological typing of oral and oropharyngeal tumours. WHO, Geneva (International histological classification of tumours, no. 4)

[2] WHO Collaborating Centre for Oral Precancerous Lesions (1978) Definition of leukoplakia and related lesions: an aid to studies on oral precancer. Oral Surg Oral Med Oral Pathol 46: 518–539

or definition. The views expressed in this volume represent those of the majority of participants with due regard to consistency with other volumes in this series.

It will, of course, be appreciated that the classification reflects the present state of knowledge, and modifications are almost certain to be needed as experience accumulates. It is therefore expected that some pathologists may wish to dissent from certain aspects of the classification or terminology adopted in this volume. It is nevertheless hoped that, in the interests of international cooperation and comparability of data, all pathologists will use the classification as put forward. Criticisms and suggestions for its improvement will be welcomed; these should be sent to the World Health Organization, Geneva, Switzerland.

The histological classification of cancer and precancer of the oral mucosa, which appears on pp. 9–10, contains the morphology code numbers of the International Classification of Diseases for Oncology (ICD-0)[1] and/or the Systematized Nomenclature of Medicine (SNOMED)[2].

The publications in the series *International Histological Classification of Tumours* are not intended to serve as textbooks but rather to promote the adoption of uniform terminology that will facilitate communication among cancer workers. For this reason literature references have been largely omitted and readers are referred to standard works for bibliographies.

Acknowledgement

Financial assistance was received from the Danish Cancer Society to enable colour photographs to be included in this monograph.

---

[1] WHO (1990) International classification of diseases for oncology. WHO, Geneva

[2] College of American Pathologists (1982) Systematized nomenclature of medicine. Chicago

Contents

Introduction   1

**Histological Classification of Cancer
and Precancer of the Oral Mucosa**   9

Definitions and Explanatory Notes   11
Carcinomas   11
Benign Lesions Capable of Microscopically Resembling
Oral Squamous Cell Carcinoma
and Oral Verrucous Carcinoma   16
Precancerous Lesions (Clinical Classification)   21
Precancerous Lesions (Histological Classification)   24
Benign Lesions Capable of Resembling
Oral Precancerous Lesions   27
Precancerous Conditions   29

TNM Classification of Lip and Oral Cavity Carcinomas .   33

Illustrations   41

Subject Index   85

Introduction

There are two major differences in concept between this volume and others in the *International Histological Classification of Tumours* series. The first of these is the inclusion of more clinical aspects than has usually been the case and the second is a concentration on a more limited range of conditions. There are several reasons for adopting this approach. With regard to both cancer and precancer of the oral mucosa, we believe it is important that general pathologists, in whose interests this volume has primarily been written, should be informed of the significance of the clinical features of the various lesions under discussion as they may on the whole be unfamiliar with them. Also, we consider it necessary to draw attention to those conditions particular to the oral tissues that may give rise to appearances which are important in differential diagnosis but can be misleading to the pathologist who does not have detailed knowledge of these tissues. On the other hand, many of the benign and malignant tumours that affect the oral tissues have been dealt with in other volumes in the series and we believe that little or no advantage would be gained by repeating them here. In particular, other volumes that will be helpful in the identification of tumours of the orofacial region include:

Odontogenic Tumours
Salivary Gland Tumours
Tumours of the Upper Respiratory Tract and Ear
Soft Tissue Tumours
Bone Tumours
Skin Tumours

So this volume covers only cancer and precancer of the oral mucosa, as opposed to all malignant and benign tumours of all oral and oropharyngeal tissues. Metastatic spread to the oral mucosa is also excluded.

The classification adopted is based largely on the histological characteristics of the tumours and is therefore concerned with morphologically identifiable cell types and patterns as seen with conventional light microscopy. The term "tumour" is used synonymously with neoplasm. Non-neoplastic lesions that clinically or morphologically resemble oral cancer or precancer are included in this classification because of their importance in differential diagnosis. The terminology adopted for individual tumours is based on their general acceptance and worldwide usage. Particularly with regard to the oral precancerous lesions and conditions, much work remains to be done to establish the behaviour and prognostic significance of their various clinical and histological appearances. We hope this publication will promote such efforts and encourage the adoption of standardized terminology and descriptions, without which further progress and comparability between different studies will be impeded.

An attempt has been made to achieve as much consistency as possible between the terminology and definitions used in this volume and those used for similar conditions described in the volumes of the series relating to other sites or tissue types.

Histological Grading

Grading of tumours of the same histological type is performed to provide some indication of their aggressiveness, which may relate in turn to prognosis or treatment. Consideration is given to the degree of cytological and architectural similarity to the presumed tissue of origin, to nuclear pleomorphism and mitotic activity, and to the histological relationship of the neoplasm to the surrounding host tissue. As the only tumour in this volume to which grading is conventionally applied is the squamous cell carcinoma, further coverage of this topic is provided in the section dealing specifically with this tumour.

TNM Classification

The anatomical extent of disease is a major factor in assessing the prognosis of carcinomas of the oral mucosa. The TNM classification, which appears on pp. 33–40, provides a uniform system for recording, reporting and comparing data in this regard[1, 2].

Adjunctive Techniques

Although this volume concentrates on the morphological features of tissues as they appear in routine, haematoxylin and eosin-stained sections, other methods for the study of tissues and cells may also contribute to an accurate identification. These include other stains employing various dyes, electron microscopy, immunocytochemistry, cytophotometry and techniques based on various aspects of molecular biology such as DNA hybridization, tissue culture and chromosomal analysis.

Techniques and methods such as exfoliative cytology, histochemistry, immunohistochemistry, image cytometry and electron microscopy have so far not provided reliable means to determine the biological behaviour of leukoplakia or oral cancer in individual patients. It is possible that studies of oncogenes, antioncogenes and cytokines (e.g. H-ras, c-myc, p53, EGFR, PDGF) may prove to be of future importance in the evaluation of prognostic features for both oral cancer and precancerous lesions.

Epidemiology and Aetiology

It has been considered necessary to include in this volume a brief review concerning the epidemiology and aetiology of cancer of the oral mucosa. This enables attention to be drawn to the heterogeneity of oral cancer in terms not only of its geogra-

---

[1] Hermanek P, Sobin LH (eds) (1992) TNM Classification of malignant tumours, 4th edn, 2nd revision. International Union Against Cancer. Springer, Berlin Heidelberg New York

[2] Beahrs O, Henson DE, Hutter RVP, Myers M (eds) (1992) Manual for staging of cancer, 4th edn. Lippincott, Philadelphia

phical and site distribution but also by clinical type and the various aetiological factors that may be involved.

Much of the published epidemiological data about oral cancer is incorporated in the broader anatomical classifications of "cancer of the head and neck" or "cancer of the buccal cavity and pharynx". Within this context it is noteworthy that estimates have been given that approximately 8 % of all cancers in men worldwide occur in the mouth and pharynx, with a corresponding estimate for women being 4 %; these amount to around 250000 new cases in men each year and 120000 in women[1].

Analysis of information from cancer registries where intraoral cancer is distinguished from cancer in other anatomical sites shows that wide geographical variations in occurrence can be seen.[2]

For example, age-standardized average incidence rates for malignant neoplasms of the lip are highest in some of the Canadian provinces, whereas those of the tongue and other parts of the mouth show their highest values in parts of France and India. There are sometimes significant differences between the incidence figures for men and women within the same anatomical site and geographical location, and time trends can be charted by comparisons over decades. In general terms there appears to be a worldwide reduction in the incidence of intraoral cancer, which is predominantly a disease of the elderly, though a few reports have recently shown stable or slightly increasing figures amongst younger men. Cancer of the lip vermilion has decreased dramatically among white men in several industrialized countries over the last few decades.

Trends in mortality from oral cancer also show variations over time by geographical region and by age and sex, though survival rates within any particular country appear to be more static. What is indisputable, however, is that small and localized lesions have a more favourable prognosis than extensive ones.

---

[1] Parkin DM, Muir CS, Läärä E (1987) Global burden of cancer. World Health Organization and International Agency for Research on Cancer Biennial Report 1986–1987. IARC, Lyon, p 11

[2] Parkin DM, Muir CS, Whelan SL, Gao YT, Ferlay J, Powell J (1992) Cancer incidence in five continents, vol 6. IARC, Lyon (IARC scientific publications, no. 120)

Only a few epidemiological studies have evaluated the prevalence of oral precancerous lesions and conditions, and it is difficult to compare them because of differences in the way populations have been sampled and in the criteria employed for their clinical and histopathological classification. Incidence data for oral precancer are available only from a very small number of studies, carried out mostly in India.

Most epidemiological data from cancer registries do not distinguish between the different types of malignant neoplasms that can affect the oral region. However, it is clear that squamous cell carcinomas comprise a large majority, probably in the region of 80%–85%. This figure varies somewhat from one part of the world to another and between studies based on cases from hospital sources.

Squamous cell carcinomas of the oral mucosa show a strong link with the use of tobacco in many different forms and with alcohol, whereas cancer of the vermilion border of the lower lip is particularly associated with exposure to sunlight. Little is known about the influence of various aetiological factors on the histological type or grade of cancer that develops. Most lower lip and intraoral squamous cell carcinomas are well differentiated and the more poorly differentiated types do not seem to have any different aetiological background that has so far been discovered. An exception to this general statement is the strong association that apparently exists between the habit of "snuff dipping" in the southeastern region of the USA and the above average occurrence there of intraoral verrucous carcinomas.

Various infective agents, such as *Candida albicans*, *Treponema pallidum*, *Herpes simplex* virus and the human papillomavirus (HPV) have been implicated to greater or lesser extent in the aetiology of oral squamous cell carcinoma and precancerous lesions. They can, of course, give rise to distinctive histological features that may signify their presence, but they do not appear to be associated with carcinomas of any particular type or grade, nor with any different prognostic characteristics. Of the precancerous conditions, oral submucous fibrosis is linked incontrovertibly with areca nut chewing in any form, whereas the aetiological factors for oral lichen planus are not well established.

Clinical Presentations of Oral Cancer (Figs. 1–5)

Clinically, almost all oral cancers, except those in the earliest stages, have two very characteristic features in the form of ulceration and an indurated margin. In different sites, however, there are certain variations.

The term cancer of the lip usually refers to cancer of the vermilion border, with that of the lower lip being much more commonly affected than the upper lip. In contrast to cancers within the oral cavity, vermilion border cancers often have their origin in a tissue which is changed due to age and ultraviolet radiation: actinic or senile keratosis and elastosis. This is characterized by narrowing of the vermilion border, which assumes a paler colour. Melanin pigment provides protection against the actinic rays, so vermilion border cancer is rarely seen among people with heavily pigmented skin. Cancer of this modified mucosa, and precancer in the form of actinic keratosis, have more similarity to carcinoma of the skin than of the oral mucosa. Also, basal cell carcinoma, which does not occur in the oral mucosa, may encroach onto the vermilion of the lip from adjacent skin.

Cancers of the labial commissures are often preceded by a nodular leukoplakia (see Sect. 3.1) which is usually associated with a candidal infection.

In the buccal mucosa the majority of cancers are located posteriorly. Often the cancer extends into the upper or lower sulcus. In some areas of southern and Southeast Asia cancer of the buccal mucosa is the most frequent location of oral cancer. This high frequency results from the widespread habit of chewing betel quid with tobacco.

Cancer of the floor of the mouth is often located in the anterior part, close to or in the midline. In advanced cases involvement of adjacent structures is common, particularly with regard to extension into the tongue. Leukoplakia or erythroplakia may also be present.

Tongue cancer may manifest itself in a variety of ways. Often it is exophytic and associated with ulceration. Sometimes a leukoplakia may be the only expression of a carcinoma. The majority of growths arise on the lateral border and the ventral surface of the anterior two-thirds of the tongue, while only around one quarter arise in the posterior third.

Palatal cancer usually develops as a rather flat swelling that later ulcerates. The tumour shows little tendency for deep growth. Reverse smokers are at high risk for palatal cancer, which usually develops as an ulcer lateral to the midline of the hard palate; it is otherwise an uncommon oral cancer.

Although the mucosa covering the gingiva and the edentulous alveolar ridge are different in their histological structure, most investigators have not distinguished between cancer of the gingiva and cancer of the alveolar ridge; they have usually used the term "gums" for both sites. Clinically, the carcinoma begins as an ulceration, often associated with a leukoplakia, on either the gingiva or the edentulous alveolar ridge. Gingival carcinomas in particular are likely to mimic inflammatory lesions.

Cancer of the vermilion border of the lower lip tends to produce cervical lymph node metastases less commonly than cancers of similar size and histology in intraoral sites. For example, cancers of the tongue and floor of the mouth, even small ones, have a high frequency of spread to cervical nodes. Lymphatic spread is usually to the ipsilateral side of the neck, but cancers located close to or extending into the midline may spread to contralateral or bilateral lymph nodes. In rare instances a lymph node metastasis in the neck is the first sign of oral cancer.

Oral cancer may cause a variety of symptoms ranging from mild to severe and either localized to the site of the tumour or, in the case of pain, referred to other sites (e.g. ear) in the head and neck region.

Histological Classification of Cancer and Precancer of the Oral Mucosa

1   Carcinomas

1.1   Squamous cell carcinoma . . . .   8070/3[a]
1.2   Verrucous carcinoma 8051/3
1.3   Basaloid squamous cell carcinoma 8094/3
1.4   Adenoid squamous cell carcinoma 8075/3
1.5   Spindle cell carcinoma 8074/3
1.6   Adenosquamous carcinoma 8560/3
1.7   Undifferentiated carcinoma 8020/3

2   Benign Lesions Capable of Microscopically Resembling Oral Squamous Cell Carcinoma (2.1–2.7) and Oral Verrucous Carcinoma (2.8–2.11)

2.1   Papillary hyperplasia   72050
2.2   Granular cell tumour 9580/0
2.3   Discoid lupus erythematosus D-3868
2.4   Median rhomboid glossitis   21400
2.5   Keratoacanthoma   72860
2.6   Necrotizing sialometaplasia   73221
2.7   Juxtaoral organ of Chievitz
2.8   Chronic hyperplastic candidiasis
2.9   Verruciform xanthoma   55300
2.10 Verruca vulgaris   76630
2.11 Condyloma acuminatum   76720

---

[a] Morphology code of the International Classification of Diseases for Oncology (ICD-O) and the Systematized Nomenclature of Medicine (SNOMED). The prefix D- indicates the Disease code of SNOMED

3   Precancerous Lesions (Clinical Classification)

3.1   Leukoplakia   72830
3.2   Erythroplakia   58530
3.3   Palatal keratosis associated with reverse smoking   72600

4   Precancerous Lesions (Histological Classification)

4.1   Squamous epithelial dysplasia   74009
4.2   Squamous cell carcinoma in situ 8070/2
4.3   Solar keratosis   72850

**5   Benign Lesions Capable of Resembling Oral
      Precancerous Lesions**

5.1   White lesions resembling leukoplakia
5.2   Red lesions resembling erythroplakia
5.3   Focal epithelial hyperplasia   72001
5.4   Reactive and regenerative atypia   69700

6   Precancerous Conditions

6.1   Sideropenic dysphagia D-6131
6.2   Lichen planus   48900
6.3   Oral submucous fibrosis   76160
6.4   Syphilis D-0182
6.5   Discoid lupus erythematosus D-3868
6.6   Xeroderma pigmentosum   74040
6.7   Epidermolysis bullosa   51550

Definitions and Explanatory Notes

1 Carcinomas

1.1 Squamous Cell Carcinoma (Figs. 6–13)

A malignant epithelial neoplasm exhibiting squamous differentiation as characterized by the formation of keratin and/or the presence of intercellular bridges.

There is essentially no difference at a microscopic level between squamous cell carcinomas arising in the oral cavity and those seen in other sites. It has been customary to grade these neoplasms in an attempt to predict their aggressiveness and hence to establish a prognosis for the patient or an indicator for the most effective treatment. This grading is generally based on the method originally described by Broders, which takes into account a subjective assessment of the degree of keratinization, cellular and nuclear pleomorphism and mitotic activity. The grades are:

Grade 1: Well differentiated (Fig. 6): Histological and cytological features closely resemble those of the squamous epithelial lining of the oral mucosa. There are varying proportions of basal and squamous cells with intercellular bridges; keratinization is a prominent feature; few mitotic figures are seen and atypical mitoses or multinucleated epithelial cells are extremely rare; nuclear and cellular pleomorphism is minimal.

Grade 2: Moderately differentiated (Fig. 7): This is a neoplasm with features intermediate between well differentiated and poorly differentiated. Compared with well-differentiated squamous cell carcinomas, these have less keratinization and more nuclear and cellular pleomorphism; there are more mitotic figures and some are abnormal in form; intercellular bridges are less conspicuous.

Grade 3: Poorly differentiated (Figs. 8, 9): Histologically and cytologically there is only a slight resemblance to the normal stratified squamous epithelium of the oral mucosa. Keratinization is rarely present and intercellular bridges are extremely scarce; mitotic activity is frequent and atypical mitoses can readily be found; cellular and nuclear pleomorphism are obvious and multinucleated cells may be frequent.

Well and moderately differentiated tumours can be grouped together as low grade, and poorly differentiated and undifferentiated tumours as high grade. When a tumour shows different grades of differentiation, the higher grade determines the final categorization.

Despite the widespread conventional use of this classification for squamous carcinomas of the oral mucosa, there appears to be only a limited relationship with either outcome or response to treatment. This may be for a variety of reasons, such as the influence of the intraoral site and the extent of the tumour on prognosis. The value of grading may be limited by: the subjective nature of assessment of various histological and cytological features; small biopsies from neoplasms that may show considerable histological heterogeneity; poor tissue preservation; reliance on tumour cell structural characteristics rather than functional ones; and evaluation of tumour cell features in isolation from those of the surrounding supporting tissues and cells.

Because histopathological grading for oral squamous cell carcinoma is subjective and since clearly defined criteria for procedures that should be followed to establish the grade of any particular example are absent, it is difficult to compare different reports on the proportion of tumours in each grade. Most observers appear to agree, however, that well-differentiated and moderately differentiated carcinomas (Grades 1 and 2) are collectively more common than poorly differentiated (Grade 3) and undifferentiated carcinomas.

Squamous cell carcinomas of the oral mucosa are no different from those elsewhere in their capacity to extend by invasion into adjacent tissues, particularly along nerves (Fig. 10). Intravascular spread is not uncommon. As much of the oral mucosa is closely related to underlying bone, tumour infiltration into bone readily occurs. This is particularly significant in respect to involvement of the inferior dental canal in the mandible, along which tumour cells may extend without outward visible signs, though often with neural symptoms.

Invasion may occur in the form of solid sheets, cords or islands of malignant cells and sometimes by dissociated individual cancer cells. The basement membrane may be more or less distinct, or completely absent. Where invasion by islands or strands of squamous cell carcinoma involves only the most superficial regions of underlying connective tissue, just beneath the basement membrane, then the term *microinvasive squamous cell carcinoma* may be applicable (Fig. 11).

Stromal tissue infiltrated by squamous cell carcinoma may show a variable degree of chronic inflammatory cell reaction and in some instances a desmoplastic response is provoked. This may make the detection of tumour cells difficult or impossible, even with the use of cell markers. Widespread dissemination through lymphatics and blood vessels also occurs.

Papillary squamous cell carcinoma is a term applied to invasive squamous cell carcinomas that have an exophytic papillary component and may clinically resemble a verrucous carcinoma (Figs. 12, 13). The invasive component may be difficult to find and serial sections or multiple samples may be required. They tend to behave more aggressively than verrucous carcinomas.

1.2 Verrucous Carcinoma (Figs. 14, 15)

A warty variant of squamous cell carcinoma characterized by a predominantly exophytic overgrowth of well-differentiated keratinizing epithelium having minimal atypia and with locally destructive pushing margins at its interface with underlying connective tissue.

The verrucous carcinoma was originally described as a distinct entity on account of its clinical and microscopic features and its mode of behaviour. Well-differentiated, hyperplastic stratified squamous epithelium is organized into bulbous rete-ridges that exhibit little or no cytological atypia or mitotic activity. There may be a significant endophytic component and the invading margin is usually below the level of the surrounding mucosa. Deep surface invaginations are filled with keratin. The advancing epithelial border is broad and the basement membrane is generally intact. There is usually a heavy inflammatory cell reaction in the adjacent connective tissue. Local destruction of connective tissue occurs in advance of the deep epithelial border. Growth is generally slow and metastatic spread occurs late, if at all. There is a view that verrucous carcinomas may become more aggressive if irradiated.

Although most verrucous carcinomas can be distinguished from squamous cell carcinomas on the basis of their mode of growth, infrequent dysplasia and absence of metastases, there are occasionally foci of conventional squamous cell carcinomas within a verrucous carcinoma. Such lesions should be classified and treated as squamous cell carcinomas. Thorough sectioning of specimens is therefore necessary to eliminate this possibility. Another hazard in diagnosis occurs when the extremely thick layers of keratin and hyperplastic epithelium are biopsied at insufficient depth to include underlying connective tissue.

The term verrucous hyperplasia describes an exophytic overgrowth of well-differentiated keratinizing epithelium that is similar to verrucous carcinoma but without the destructive, pushing border at its interface with the underlying connective tissue. Areas of verrucous hyperplasia may be encountered in association with verrucous carcinoma, squamous cell carcinoma or proliferative verrucous leukoplakia (see Sect. 3.1).

Exophytic papillary lesions that show epithelial dysplasia, possibly even carcinoma in situ, and relatively inconspicuous areas of invasive squamous cell carcinoma separate from the surface epithelium, should be distinguished from verrucous carcinomas and classified as papillary squamous cell carcinomas (see Sect. 1.1).

1.3 Basaloid Squamous Cell Carcinoma (Figs. 16, 17)

A form of carcinoma with a mixed composition of basaloid and squamous cells.

This is a form of oral carcinoma in which the basaloid component comprises small cells with hyperchromatic nuclei and scant cytoplasm that are crowded together into lobulated sheets or strands focally connected to the surface epithelium. Cells at the periphery of the lobules are often palisaded; more centrally there may be cystic spaces, sometimes containing material resembling mucin, and focal squamous differentiation. Mitotic figures, including abnormal forms, and areas of necrosis are commonly seen. There is often hyalinization of the surrounding stroma and chronic inflammatory cell infiltration is variable. Confusion with ameloblastoma and adenoid cystic carcinoma is to be avoided; a focal squamous cell carcinoma component among the basaloid areas is the most important distinguishing feature. Most cases have been described in the larynx, hypopharynx and base of the tongue.

1.4 Adenoid Squamous Cell Carcinoma (Figs. 18, 19)

A squamous cell carcinoma containing pseudoglandular spaces or lumina.

This variant is produced as a result of acantholysis and degeneration within islands of a squamous cell carcinoma. The result is a pseudoadenocarcinomatous appearance, but there is no evidence of glandular differentiation or of secretory activity or products. There are insufficient reported cases to establish likely behaviour.

1.5 Spindle Cell Carcinoma (Fig. 20)

A carcinoma within which there are some elements resembling a squamous cell carcinoma that are associated with a spindle cell component.

In a true spindle cell carcinoma the malignant spindle-shaped cells should be demonstrably of epithelial origin and derived from the squamous cell component of the carcinoma. This must be distinguished both from a squamous cell carcinoma that has provoked a reactive fibroblastic stromal proliferation and from a carcinosarcoma in which a squamous cell carcinoma is accompanied by a sarcoma of fibroblastic or other connective tissue cell type. Care should also be taken not to confuse a spindle cell carcinoma with a spindle cell malignant melanoma or with sarcomas of various types.

Often the squamous cell carcinoma component in a spindle cell carcinoma is inconspicuous and multiple sections or blocks may be necessary to find it. Most of the neoplasm comprises thin elongated cells amongst which there may be occasional pleomorphic cells. Mitotic figures, including abnormal forms, are usually not difficult to find. Behaviour is similar to that of the more frequent and usual type of squamous cell carcinoma.

1.6 Adenosquamous Carcinoma (Fig. 21)

A malignant tumour with histological features of both adenocarcinoma and squamous cell carcinoma.

This tumour may arise from the ducts of minor salivary glands or from the overlying surface epithelium. The component identified as squamous cell carcinoma may be in situ or invasive, and the adenocarcinomatous component comprises glandular structures lined by basaloid, columnar or mucin-secreting cells. Distinction between adenosquamous carcinoma and high-grade mucoepidermoid carcinoma may be difficult, though in the former the glandular and squamous components are generally more distinct. Care must also be taken to distinguish adenosquamous carcinoma from adenoid squamous cell carcinoma.

1.7 Undifferentiated Carcinoma (Fig. 22)

A carcinoma that lacks evidence of squamous, glandular or other types of differentiation.

Accurate diagnosis is almost certainly dependent upon the use of adjunctive diagnostic techniques.

2 Benign Lesions Capable of Microscopically Resembling Oral Squamous Cell Carcinoma (2.1–2.7) and Oral Verrucous Carcinoma (2.8–2.11)

2.1 Papillary Hyperplasia (Figs. 23–25)

Papillary hyperplasia is a benign overgrowth of the mucosa and is almost exclusively seen on the hard palate of denture-wearing patients. Clinically, the lesion is composed of small, soft, sessile, papillary projections, which are usually bright red in colour.

Histologically, the epithelium is folded and thickened and may show pseudoepitheliomatous hyperplasia. Subepithelial oedema and infiltration by chronic inflammatory cells is common and fibrosis of connective tissue papillae may be seen in long-standing cases. In some instances candidal hyphae are present in the superficial layers of the epithelium.

A small biopsy might be histologically misdiagnosed as a carcinoma.

2.2 Granular Cell Tumour (Fig. 26)

The granular cell tumour, a benign soft tissue lesion of probable neurogenic type, is included in this classification of oral mucosal lesions because of the pseudoepitheliomatous hyperplasia that frequently overlies the tumour. A superficial biopsy that includes few or no underlying granular cells may easily be misinterpreted as a squamous cell carcinoma.

2.3 Discoid Lupus Erythematosus (Figs. 27, 28)

Lupus erythematosus (LE) is a chronic autoimmune disorder of unknown aetiology. The discoid type of LE is characterized by skin involvement, particularly of the face, and in some cases oral manifestations are seen. Clinically, oral discoid lesions are characterized by central atrophy, small white keratinized plaques with elevated borders, radiating white striae, and telangiectasia. In some instances pseudoepitheliomatous changes can be misdiagnosed as squamous cell carcinoma. Oral carcinoma may arise in the atrophied epithelium (see Sect. 6.5).

The histological features may resemble to some extent the features of lichen planus. There may be slight parakeratosis or hyperkeratosis, keratin horn plugs, hydropic degeneration of the basal cell layer, degeneration of the collagen in the underlying connective tissue, and a predominantly lymphocytic infiltrate which tends to be located perivascularly.

2.4 Median Rhomboid Glossitis (Figs. 29, 30)

Median rhomboid glossitis is a benign lesion clinically characterized by a red, usually smooth, sometimes slightly elevated and lobulated, appearance of the lingual mucosa just anterior to the foramen caecum. Its size may vary from a few millimeters to a few centimeters in diameter. *Candida albicans* infection appears to play a role in its aetiology. The lesion is mostly observed in adults.

It is almost always justified to diagnose median rhomboid glossitis on the basis of clinical appearance, without the need for histopathological confirmation. Squamous cell carcinoma of the tongue rarely arises in the midline of the dorsum, but a superficial biopsy of median rhomboid glossitis may be mistaken for squamous cell carcinoma due to the irregular pattern of the rete-ridges and occasional presence of pseudoepitheliomatous hyperplasia. Signs of epithelial dysplasia are absent, as is mitotic activity. A hyperparakeratinized surface layer and chronic inflammatory cell infiltration of subepithelial connective tissue are characteristic.

2.5 Keratoacanthoma (Figs. 31, 32)

The keratoacanthoma, also called molluscum sebaceum, is a cutaneous lesion that is believed to arise from hair follicles through a viral infection. It is generally considered to be benign. Occurrence on the lower lip is uncommon, and an intraoral location is exceptionally rare.

It is a solitary, rapidly growing, well-circumscribed, slightly elevated lesion that rarely measures more than 1 cm in diameter. Centrally, a keratin-filled crater with slightly indurated borders can be seen. Clinically, the lesion may mimic a squamous cell carcinoma, but it enlarges more rapidly and involution occurs spontaneously within 2–6 months.

Histologically, the lesion appears as a raised hemispherical mass in the dermis composed of a central plug of keratin surrounded by nests and columns of stratified squamous epithelium. There is limited pushing infiltration at the stromal interface that seldom extends below the level of the sweat glands. A chronic inflammatory cell reaction is typically present at the periphery. The epidermis covering the lesion dips into the sides of

the central keratin-filled crater. The lesion may exhibit cytological atypia, dyskeratosis and mitotic activity. It is distinguished
from squamous cell carcinoma by its clinical features and by its
overall architecture; the latter, however, may not be evident in
biopsies that do not include the central crater, base and margins
of the lesion. Many carcinomas of the lip vermilion have features similar to those of the keratoacanthoma.

2.6 Necrotizing Sialometaplasia (Figs. 33, 34)

This is an ischaemic lesion mostly localized in the palate. The
term "salivary gland infarction" is sometimes used, based on
the fact that the lesion resembles infarcts in other organs, such
as the prostate gland. Necrotizing sialometaplasia may follow
ischaemia or trauma (including recent surgical procedures) and
resolves spontaneously. The initial clinical presentation is often
a mucosal nodule that soon shows secondary ulceration of the
surface.

Histologically, the lesion shows lobular necrosis of salivary
gland acini and squamous cell metaplasia of the duct system in
the centre. Mitoses are not uncommon. Inflammatory cell infiltration is found peripherally. These features are usually surrounded by intact glandular tissue. Pseudoepitheliomatous hyperplasia may also be observed.

The lesion can usually be distinguished from squamous cell
carcinoma and mucoepidermoid carcinoma by the preservation
of the lobular architecture of the necrotic glandular cells.

2.7 Juxtaoral Organ of Chievitz (Fig. 35)

The organ of Chievitz occurs in the buccotemporal space. The
true nature of these juxtaoral organs is unknown; possibly they
represent rudimentary or atavistic structures. Juxtaoral organs
may histologically be misinterpreted as squamous cell carcinoma
and perineural carcinomatous spread. They comprise small
ovoid or rounded nests of squamous cells, sometimes with basal
cell palisading, associated with fine nerve fibres. The localiza-
tion, the characteristic organization of the connective tissue,
and the relation of the organs to branches of the buccal nerve
are usually sufficient for diagnosis.

2.8 Chronic Hyperplastic Candidiasis (Figs. 36–38)

The presence of *C. albicans* can be demonstrated in about one-third of the population as shown by culturing smears or swabs from apparently healthy oral mucosa. Fungal overgrowth or invasion of the tissues produces clinically visible lesions referred to as candidiasis.

Candidiasis can be classified into different types, such as pseudomembranous, erythematous, and chronic mucocutaneous. In some lesions it is questionable whether the presence of *C. albicans* in the tissues is a primary cause or a secondary phenomenon. This is particularly true in hyperplastic candidiasis. Some authors prefer the term "candidal leukoplakia" or "*Candida*-associated leukoplakia" rather than hyperplastic candidiasis in such cases, particularly for lesions occurring in the labial commissures and on the dorsum of the tongue.

Histologically, hyperplastic candidiasis is characterized by parakeratotic hyperplastic epithelium that is invaded superficially by candidal hyphae; these can be demonstrated by a periodic acid-Schiff (PAS) stain. Inflammatory cells may be present throughout the entire thickness of the epithelium and often form polymorphonuclear leukocyte microabscesses in the superficial layer. The rete-ridges may be broad, mimicking to some extent the architecture of a verrucous carcinoma. There is often a diffuse infiltrate of lymphocytes and plasma cells in the lamina propria.

2.9 Verruciform Xanthoma (Figs. 39, 40)

The verruciform xanthoma is a rare lesion of the oral mucosa and skin. Its aetiology is unknown. Clinically, the lesion presents as a red, yellow-red or grey, somewhat pedunculated and sharply demarcated nodule or plaque. Histological examination shows a papillomatous epithelial surface with hyperkeratosis and numerous histiocyte-like foam cells in the connective tissue papillae. It has been suggested that degenerative changes in the epithelium primarily lead to the presence of the foam cells. Although usually comparatively small in size, the verruciform xanthoma could be mistaken for an early squamous cell or verrucous carcinoma.

2.10 Verruca Vulgaris (Figs. 41, 42)

This is the oral counterpart of the lesion seen more commonly on the skin and caused by HPV types 2 and 4.

The squamous epithelium typically shows papillomatosis, acanthosis and variable hyperkeratosis, primarily of the parakeratotic type. It often has a prominent granular layer with cells containing large keratohyaline granules and cells with pyknotic nuclei surrounded by a halo of clear cytoplasm ("koilocytes") in the superficial layers. The rete-ridges at the periphery of the lesion are usually bent inwards towards the centre. If tangentially cut, a verruca vulgaris may resemble early well-differentiated squamous cell carcinoma.

2.11 Condyloma Acuminatum

Condyloma acuminatum (venereal wart) occurs most frequently on anogenital skin and mucosa and is caused by HPV.

Several cases of intraoral occurrence have been reported, caused by oro-genital contact. These are largely associated with HPV types 6 and 11.

Histologically, the lesions show hyperplastic epithelium arranged in a papillomatous pattern, mostly without keratinization. There is often vacuolization of the epithelial cells of the spinous cell layer and koilocytes are frequently seen.

3 Precancerous Lesions
(Clinical Classification)

A morphologically altered tissue in which cancer is more likely to occur than in its apparently normal counterpart.

3.1 Leukoplakia (Figs. 43–47)

A predominantly white lesion of the oral mucosa that cannot be characterized as any other definable lesion.

Over the years the term leukoplakia has been used for lesions having a whitish appearance as the common denominator and some of which have proved to be precancerous. Studies have shown that such whitish lesions may have widely different aetiological backgrounds, which may be related to their malignant potential.

Whitish patches or plaques for which a local cause can be identified should be classified according to the established cause and not be included among leukoplakias. Examples are lesions associated with friction, dental restorations, cheek-biting, and glassblowing (see below). Lesions with a white appearance that cannot be clearly diagnosed on clinical examination as any other disease of the oral mucosa should be provisionally diagnosed as oral leukoplakia. A definitive diagnosis of oral leukoplakia is made as a result of the identification, and if possible elimination, of suspected aetiological factors and, in the case of persistent lesions, histopathological examination.

The term "hairy leukoplakia" has recently been introduced to describe a characteristic white lesion that almost exclusively occurs bilaterally on the borders of the tongue in some HIV-infected individuals. This terminology is potentially misleading as it does not coincide with the definition of leukoplakia (as given above) and in itself carries no risk of malignant transformation.

According to their *clinical* appearance, leukoplakias may be classified as either homogeneous or non-homogeneous. The latter comprise about 10 % of all leukoplakias. Table 1 gives a classification based upon clinical criteria.

Homogeneous leukoplakias may be found in all regions of the oral mucosa. The lesion is white or whitish with a surface that may be flat, corrugated, cracked, wrinkled, or pumice-like.

The corrugated type is especially found in the floor of the mouth, and is sometimes called the "ebbing-tide" type of leukoplakia. The anatomical location of the lesion may influence its morphology.

Wrinkling of the mucosal surface is characteristic of the type seen only in individuals using snuff intraorally. The intensity of

Table 1. Clinical classification of leukoplakias

Homogeneous leukoplakias	*Non-homogeneous leukoplakias*
Flat	Verrucous
Corrugated	Nodular
Wrinkled	Ulcerated
Pumice-like	Erythroleukoplakia

wrinkling has been used in grading the severity of the lesions in studies in Sweden and the USA. The openings of minor salivary gland ducts on the surface may be present as red punctate features. This type only very rarely exhibits dysplasia.

The fourth type of homogeneous leukoplakia is the pumice-like type. It is characterized by delicate white striae and appears to be a specific reaction of the oral mucosa that may be caused either by smoking tobacco or by snuff usage.

Often a mixed pattern of the above clinical types may be observed.

Non-homogeneous leukoplakias may also be found on any oral mucosal surface. They are predominantly white with verrucous, nodular, ulcerated or erythematous features and are more dangerous when found to be indurated on palpation. In general terms, they present a greater risk of malignant change than the homogeneous types. The verrucous type is characterized by a warty appearance and may be difficult to distinguish from squamous papilloma or verrucous carcinoma. A rare type is characterized by being multifocal, slow growing and with a propensity to recur after excision. Some have described this type as *proliferative verrucous leukoplakia*; in the past it has sometimes been called oral florid papillomatosis. Nearly all cases of proliferative verrucous leukoplakia eventually undergo malignant transformation at multiple sites. The nodular type of leukoplakia, originally described as speckled leukoplakia, possesses the important clinical feature of white nodular excrescences. In between the predominating nodules, the mucosa is often erythematous (erythroleukoplakia).

A homogeneous leukoplakia that becomes infected with *C. albicans*, which is often the case, may change its clinical appearance and become ulcerated or more erythematous. Such a lesion may eventually develop into a nodular leukoplakia. Non-homogeneous leukoplakias treated with local antifungal agents may correspondingly revert to the homogeneous type.

The term erythroleukoplakia is used when a lesion is composed of a mixture of white areas, often in the form of white nodules, and red areas.

3.2 Erythroplakia (Fig. 48)

A fiery red patch that cannot be characterized clinically or pathologically as any other definable lesion.

Some erythroplakias are smooth and some are granular or nodular. Often there is a well-defined margin adjacent to mucosa of normal appearance. The soft palate, ventral surface of the tongue and floor of the mouth are the most likely sites to be involved, but any part of the oral mucosa may be affected. Erythroplakias are high-risk lesions for the subsequent development of carcinoma.

3.3 Palatal Keratosis Associated with Reverse Smoking (Fig. 49)

A diffuse whitening of the palatal mucosa in reverse smokers.

This occurs with or without the following features: elevated white patches, red areas, ulcerations and hyper-pigmented or non-pigmented areas. In several countries cigars or cigarettes are smoked with the glowing end inside the mouth. The largest number of reverse smokers is found in certain areas of India, but the habit is also practised in some Latin American countries, in Sardinia and in the Philippines.

4 Precancerous Lesions
(Histological Classification)

Although leukoplakia is a clinical term and its use carries no implications with regard to histological findings, a histological report should always include a statement on the presence or absence of epithelial dysplasia and, if present, an assessment of its severity. Sometimes malignancy develops in association with an oral leukoplakia for which earlier biopsies have not demonstrated epithelial dysplasia.

The majority of homogeneous leukoplakias show hyperorthokeratosis and acanthosis (Fig. 50) without signs of epithelial dysplasia. Inflammation may or may not be present in the lamina propria.

Those leukoplakias that are not hyperorthokeratotic exhibit hyperparakeratosis (Fig.51). The mitotic activity of hyperparakeratotic leukoplakias is usually higher than in the hyperorthokeratotic types but this, by itself, should not be interpreted as a sign of dysplasia. Characteristically, hyperparakeratotic lesions usually have a much thicker epithelium than those with hyperorthokeratosis.

A special form of hyperkeratinization is the so-called chevron type of parakeratosis that is confined to non-keratinized oral mucosa (Fig.52) and seems to be a specific reaction of the oral mucosa to tobacco. It is characterized by streaks of parakeratosis with a chevron-like pattern. The streaks are often raised beyond the adjacent layers, giving the surface a fingerprint-like appearance clinically.

Non-homogeneous leukoplakias are often associated with epithelial dysplasia, carcinoma in situ or squamous cell carcinoma. The same is true for erythroplakias and erythroleukoplakias.

4.1 Squamous Epithelial Dysplasia (Figs.53–55)

A precancerous lesion of stratified squamous epithelium characterized by cellular atypia and loss of normal maturation and stratification short of carcinoma in situ.

The general disturbance of the epithelium is designated dysplasia and the potential for developing invasive carcinoma increases with the severity of dysplasia.

The changes that may occur in epithelial dysplasia are listed in Table 2, and the more prominent or more numerous they are, the more severe the grade of dysplasia. It will, of course, be appreciated that not all these changes are necessarily seen in any one case and that there is considerable subjectivity involved in their recognition and the interpretation of their significance in various combinations and forms. It should also be noted that some cellular atypia, usually of minor degree, is often present in inflammatory conditions and in regenerating epithelium. Sometimes epithelial dysplasia may be seen in lichen planus and in candidiasis.

The relationship of epithelial dysplasia in its various grades (commonly divided into mild, moderate and severe) to the subsequent development of cancer has not been fully clarified. However, it is generally believed that any degree of epithelial

Table 2. Histological changes that may contribute to a diagnosis of epithelial dysplasia

---

Loss of polarity of the basal cells

The presence of more than one layer having a basaloid appearance

Increased nuclear-cytoplasmic ratio

Drop-shaped rete-ridges

Irregular epithelial stratification

Increased number of mitotic figures

Mitotic figures that are abnormal in form

The presence of mitotic figures in the superficial half of the epithelium

Cellular and nuclear pleomorphism

Nuclear hyperchromatism

Enlarged nucleoli

Loss of intercellular adherence

Keratinization of single cells or cell groups in the prickle cell layer

---

dysplasia, even a mild form, indicates an increased risk for the patient. Severe dysplasia indicates that there is a very high risk of the subsequent development of cancer. Dysplasia is often seen co-existing with invasive carcinoma.

4.2 Squamous Cell Carcinoma In Situ (Fig. 56)

A lesion in which the full thickness, or almost the full thickness, of squamous epithelium shows the cellular features of carcinoma without stromal invasion.

Severe grades of epithelial dysplasia may merge into the lesion customarily designated as carcinoma in situ, in which the whole, or almost the whole, thickness of the epithelium is involved. However, distinguishing between severe dysplasia and carcinoma in situ is often difficult and does not appear to be of practical value in the case of the oral mucosa. In the present state of knowledge it is not possible to say whether severe epithelial dysplasia carries a different degree of risk of subsequent development of invasive carcinoma than that associated with carcinoma in situ.

4.3 Solar Keratosis (Actinic Keratosis)

Epidermal dysplasia due to actinic radiation.

The squamous epithelium of the lip vermilion may be hyperplastic or atrophic and shows disordered maturation, varying degrees of keratinization, cytological atypia and increased mitotic activity. Keratin may accumulate to form a surface plaque. The underlying connective tissue usually shows basophilic degeneration of collagen and elastosis. Squamous cell carcinoma often develops in untreated cases.

5 Benign Lesions Capable of Resembling Oral Precancerous Lesions

5.1 White Lesions Resembling Leukoplakia
(Figs. 57–70)

Histologically, lesions in this category, such as those mentioned in the following sections, show a variable degree or type of keratosis, acanthosis and epithelial hyperplasia; there may be ballooning, vacuolization or spongiosis of the prickle cells and pyknosis of nuclei. However, the changes are insufficient to warrant categorization as epithelial dysplasia. The extent of any cellular infiltrate in the supporting connective tissue is also variable.

Lesions that are sometimes similar in appearance to leukoplakia or lichen planus may occasionally be associated with restorative materials; for example, in areas of the oral mucosa in close contact with corroded amalgam restorations. In some of these lesions there is a superimposed candidal infection.

Frictional lesions are most often observed on the margin and alveolar part of the gingiva and are caused by inexpedient toothbrushing. Together with the white lesion there may be cervical abrasion of the involved teeth and gingival recession. Glassblower lesions, most likely due to heat, represent another type of highly reversible white patch.

Various other lesions may present clinically as solid white or whitish areas or plaques on the oral mucosa; these include morsicatio buccarum (cheek biting), leukoedema, aspirin burn, white sponge naevus, lichen planus, hairy leukoplakia and pseudomembranous candidiasis (thrush).

5.2 Red Lesions Resembling Erythroplakia
(Figs. 71–73)

In some patients chronic erythematous candidiasis may resemble an erythroplakia. However, in this form of candidiasis the erythematous area is always on a level with the adjacent mucosa. Most cases of erythematous candidiasis are located on either the mucosa of the palate or dorsum of the tongue – areas where it is unusual to find erythroplakia.

One of the six clinical types of oral lichen planus is characterized by a red, well-circumscribed area; this is called atrophic lichen planus. Distinguishing atrophic lichen planus from erythroplakia may be difficult as approximately 1 % of oral lichen planus cases are associated with a simultaneous erythroplakia. A biopsy is desirable in cases of doubt.

Areas of reddened oral mucosa that may simulate erythroplakia also include various types of mucositis associated with infections, such as tuberculosis and histoplasmosis, and with a range of miscellaneous conditions that includes pemphigoid and the palatal erythema associated with bidi smoking.

5.3 Focal Epithelial Hyperplasia (Figs. 74–76)

Focal epithelial hyperplasia is characterized by multiple papules, plaques, or swellings of the oral mucosa. It is mainly a children's disease and in some of the reported cases there is a distinct familial occurrence.

The clinical presentation is a non-painful wart-like lesion that may form aggregates with adjacent lesions. The colour of the papules is usually the same as that of the surrounding mucosa. In most cases the diagnosis can reliably be made based on clinical aspects only.

Histologically, hyperplasia of the stratum spinosum results in thickening and lengthening of the rete-ridges, which may show some clubbing and/or fusion. The upper epithelial layers may contain mitotic-like figures ("mitosoid cells") which can be misinterpreted as epithelial dysplasia or, if sufficiently numerous, carcinoma in situ. Subepithelially, a slight inflammatory infiltrate may be encountered. Ultrastructural examination has demonstrated the presence of virus-like particles in the epithelium, and in situ hybridization demonstrates specific viral DNA.

The lesions do not require therapy and carry no premalignant connotation. Spontaneous regression occurs in some cases.

5.4 Reactive and Regenerative Atypia (Fig. 77)

Cellular atypia and proliferation of immature squamous epithelium occur in response to a variety of injurious, inflammatory and ulcerative lesions. For example, ionizing radiation can produce marked cytological changes. Pseudoepitheliomatous hyperplasia adjacent to chronic ulcers may show sufficient atypia to mimic dysplasia. Furthermore, bizarre, yet benign, reactive stromal cells may populate the granulation tissue of an ulcer. Rebiopsy after a suitable interval will usually help to resolve the nature of such changes.

6 Precancerous Conditions

A generalized state associated with a significantly increased risk of cancer.

Examples of precancerous conditions are sideropenic dysphagia, oral submucous fibrosis, syphilis, discoid lupus erythematosus and xeroderma pigmentosum. Apart from these, consideration must be given to more generalized diseases, such as lichen planus, that make the mucosa more susceptible to carcinogens and thus to the development of oral cancer.

The common histological denominator for precancerous conditions is epithelial atrophy, which is characteristic of the diseases described below.

6.1 Sideropenic Dysphagia

Sideropenic dysphagia (Paterson–Kelly or Plummer–Vinson syndrome) mainly affects middle-aged women, with iron deficiency being the underlying cause. The entire oral mucosa is red, shiny and atrophic. Leukoplakias as well as multiple oral carcinomas may develop, predominantly in the posterior part of the mouth and in the oropharynx.

6.2 Lichen Planus (Figs. 65, 66, 72, 73)

Lichen planus is an inflammatory disease of skin and mucosa of unknown aetiology, though alterations in cell-mediated immunity may be important. Clinically, six types of oral lichen planus are described: papular, reticular, plaque-like, atrophic, erosive (ulcerative) and bullous. Malignant transformation has been observed in up to 2%–3% of patients in a number of studies. Female patients with lichen planus were found to show a 50-fold increase in oral cancer compared with the expected rate of oral cancer development in a sample of the general population of comparable gender and age distribution.

Histologically, oral lichen planus is characterized by hyperkeratosis, either of an ortho- or para-keratinization type, acanthosis or epithelial atrophy, basal cell liquefaction degeneration, a subepithelial eosinophilic amorphous band, and a dense, well-defined infiltrate of lymphocytes in the superficial lamina propria. Epithelial rete-ridges are frequently missing or may have a "saw-tooth" appearance. Dysplastic changes are sometimes seen.

6.3 Oral Submucous Fibrosis (Figs. 78–80)

Oral submucous fibrosis is characterized by epithelial atrophy and fibrosis of the subepithelial connective tissue, resulting in stiffness of the oral mucosa. Leukoplakia may be superimposed. There is convincing epidemiological and other evidence from the populations of southern and Southeast Asia that areca nut chewing is the principal aetiological agent; however, genetic traits have also been suspected as predisposing factors in some cases.

Histologically, oral submucous fibrosis is characterized by severe epithelial atrophy and an underlying dense collagenous tissue with coarse fibre formation. Varying degrees of hyperkeratosis and epithelial dysplasia may also be present. Oral submucous fibrosis predisposes to the development of oral cancer.

6.4 Syphilis

Leukoplakic lesions may develop in the atrophic epithelium associated with the glossitis often seen in tertiary syphilis. In later stages the leukoplakia may undergo malignant transformation.

6.5 Discoid Lupus Erythematosus

Oral lesions in discoid lupus erythematosus may show pseudo-epitheliomatous hyperplasia and consequently are described in Sect. 2.3. Classification here with other precancerous conditions is necessary because a few cases of squamous cell carcinoma developing in discoid lupus erythematosus have been reported, especially in atrophied epithelium on the vermilion border of the lower lip.

6.6 Xeroderma Pigmentosum

Xeroderma pigmentosum is a neurocutaneous disease with a recessive mode of inheritance. The lips are mainly affected and show epithelial atrophy, telangiectasia and hyperpigmentation, which may occasionally also be observed on the oral mucosa. Squamous cell carcinoma of the oral mucosa has been observed in some affected individuals.

6.7 Epidermolysis Bullosa

Epidermolysis bullosa, particularly the dystrophic type, is an inherited disorder of either autosomal dominant or recessive pattern. The disease is characterized by formation of bullae of the skin and oral mucosa. Oral scarring results in loss of the oral vestibulum, ankyloglossia and microstomia. Carcinoma of the tongue has been described in cases of dystrophic epidermolysis bullosa.

TNM Classification of Lip and Oral Cavity Carcinomas[1]

Rules for Classification

The classification applies only to carcinomas of the vermilion surfaces of the lips and of the oral cavity, including those of minor salivary glands. There should be histological confirmation of the disease. The following are the procedures for assessment of the T,N and M categories:

T categories   Physical examination and imaging
N categories   Physical examination and imaging
M categories   Physical examination and imaging

Anatomical Sites and Subsites

Lip

1. External upper lip (vermilion border) (C00.0)
2. External lower lip (vermilion border) (C00.1)
3. Commissures (C00.6)

Oral Cavity

1. Buccal mucosa
   i)   Mucosa of upper and lower lips (C00.3,4)
   ii) Cheek mucosa (C06.0)
   iii) Retromolar areas (C06.2)
   iv) Bucco-alveolar sulci, upper and lower (vestibule of mouth) (C06.1)
2. Upper alveolus and gingiva (upper gum) (C03.0)
3. Lower alveolus and gingiva (lower gum) (C03.1)

---

[1] Hermanek P, Sobin LH (eds) (1992) TNM Classification of malignant tumours, 4th edn, 2nd revision. International Union Against Cancer. Springer, Berlin Heidelberg New York

4. Hard palate (C05.0)
5. Tongue
   i) Dorsal surface and lateral borders anterior to vallate pa-
       pillae (anterior two-thirds) (C02.0,1)
   ii) Inferior (ventral) surface (C02.2)
6. Floor of mouth (C04)

Regional Lymph Nodes

The regional lymph nodes are the cervical nodes.

TNM Clinical Classification

T – Primary Tumour

TX Primary tumour cannot be assessed
T0 No evidence of primary tumour
Tis Carcinoma in situ
T1 Tumour 2 cm or less in greatest dimension
T2 Tumour more than 2 cm but not more than 4 cm in greatest
    dimension
T3 Tumour more than 4 cm in greatest dimension
T4 *Lip:* Tumour invades adjacent structures, e.g. through cor-
    tical bone, tongue, skin of neck
    Oral cavity: Tumour invades adjacent structures, e.g.
    through cortical bone, into deep (extrinsic) muscle of ton-
    gue, maxillary sinus, skin

N – Regional Lymph Nodes

NX Regional lymph nodes cannot be assessed
N0 No regional lymph node metastasis
N1 Metastasis in a single ipsilateral lymph node, 3 cm or less
    in greatest dimension
N2 Metastasis in a single ipsilateral lymph node, more than
    3 cm but not more than 6 cm in greatest dimension, or in
    multiple ipsilateral lymph nodes, none more than 6 cm in
    greatest dimension, or in bilateral or contralateral lymph
    nodes, none more than 6 cm in greatest dimension
    N2a Metastasis in a single ipsilateral lymph node, more
         than 3 cm but not more than 6 cm in greatest dimen-
         sion
    N2b Metastasis in multiple ipsilateral lymph nodes, none
         more than 6 cm in greatest dimension

N2c Metastasis in bilateral or contralateral lymph nodes, none more than 6 cm in greatest dimension

N3 Metastasis in a lymph node, more than 6 cm in greatest dimension

Note: Midline nodes are considered ipsilateral nodes

M – Distant Metastasis

MX Presence of distant metastasis cannot be assessed
M0 No distant metastasis
M1 Distant metastasis

pTNM Pathological Classification

The pT, pN and pM categories correspond to the T, N and M categories.

Stage Grouping

Stage 0	Tis	N0	M0
Stage I	T1	N0	M0
Stage II	T2	N0	M0
Stage III	T1	N1	M0
	T2	N1	M0
	T3	N0,N1	M0
Stage IV	T4	N0, N1	M0
	Any T	N2,N3	M0
	Any T	Any N	M1

Summary

Lip, Oral Cavity	
T1	< 2 cm
T2	> 2–4 cm
T3	> 4 cm
T4	Adjacent structures
N1	Ipsilateral single ≤ 3 cm
N2	Ipsilateral single > 3–6 cm
	Ipsilateral multiple ≤ 6 cm
	Bilateral, contralateral ≤ 6 cm
N3	> 6 cm

TN Clinical Classification[1]

T – Primary Tumour

TX   Primary tumour cannot be assessed
T0   No evidence of primary tumour
Tis Carcinoma in situ
T1   Tumour 2 cm or less in greatest dimension
T2   Tumour more than 2 cm but not more than 4 cm in greatest
     dimension
T3   Tumour more than 4 cm in greatest dimension (see p. 37)

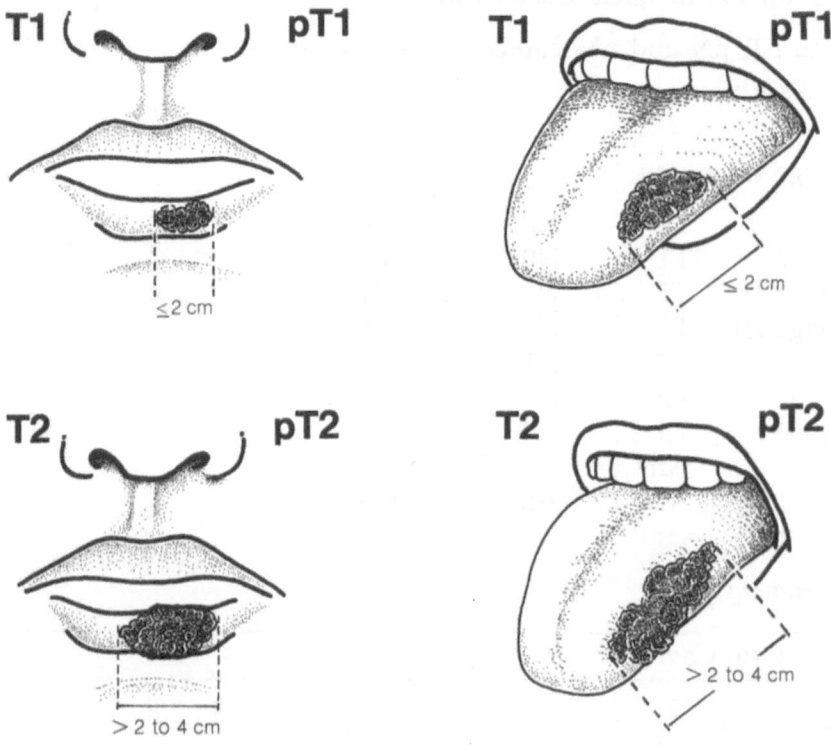

___

[1] The figures on pp 36–40 are reproduced from Spiessl B, Beahrs OH, Hermanek P, Hutter RVP, Scheibe O, Sobin LH, Wagner G (eds) (1992) TNM atlas.
Illustrated guide to the TNM/pTNM classification of malignant tumours, 3rd
edn, 2nd revision. Springer, Berlin Heidelberg New York, pp 4 and 14–17

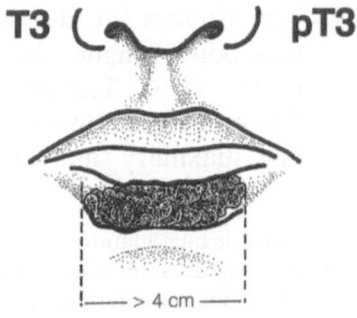

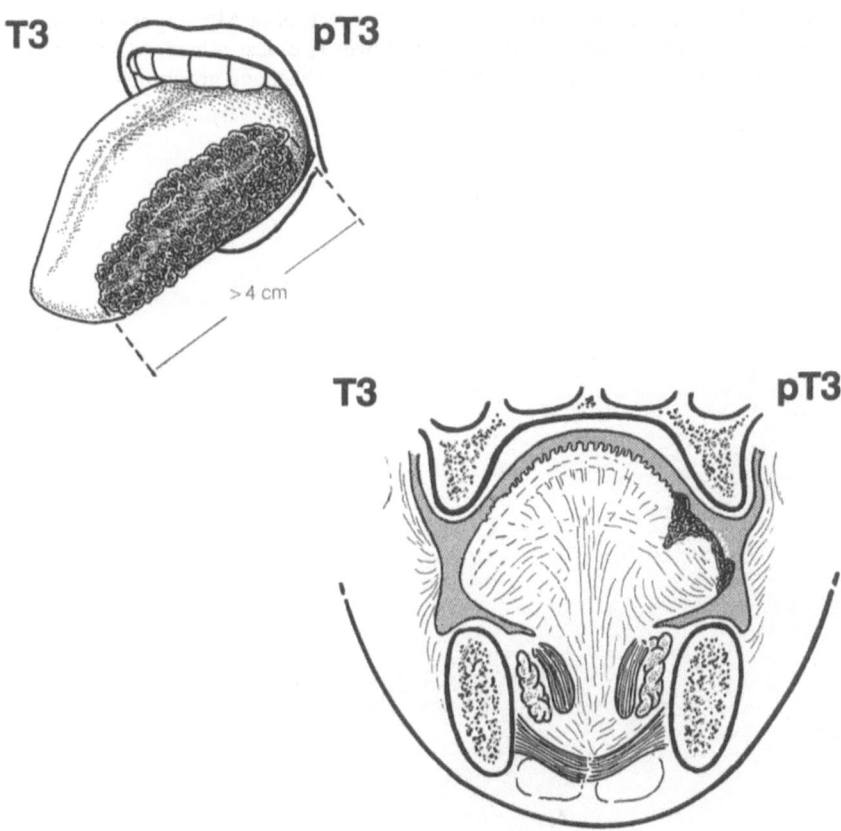

T4   *Lip*: Tumour invades adjacent structures, e.g. through cortical bone, tongue, skin of neck
Oral cavity: Tumour invades adjacent structures, e.g. through cortical bone, into deep (extrinsic) muscle of tongue, maxillary sinus, skin

Notes:

1. The *extrinsic* musculature of the tongue includes musculi hyo-, stylo-, genio- and palatoglossus. Invasion of the *intrinsic muscle alone* (musculi longitudinales superior and inferior, transversus linguae and verticalis linguae) is not classified T4.
2. In cases of doubt regarding the invasion through cortical bone, paragraph 4 of the General Rules of the TNM System (TNM Booklet, p. 6) should be applied: "If there is doubt concerning the correct T, N or M category to which a particular case should be allotted, the lower (i.e. less advanced) category should be chosen. This will also be reflected in the stage grouping".

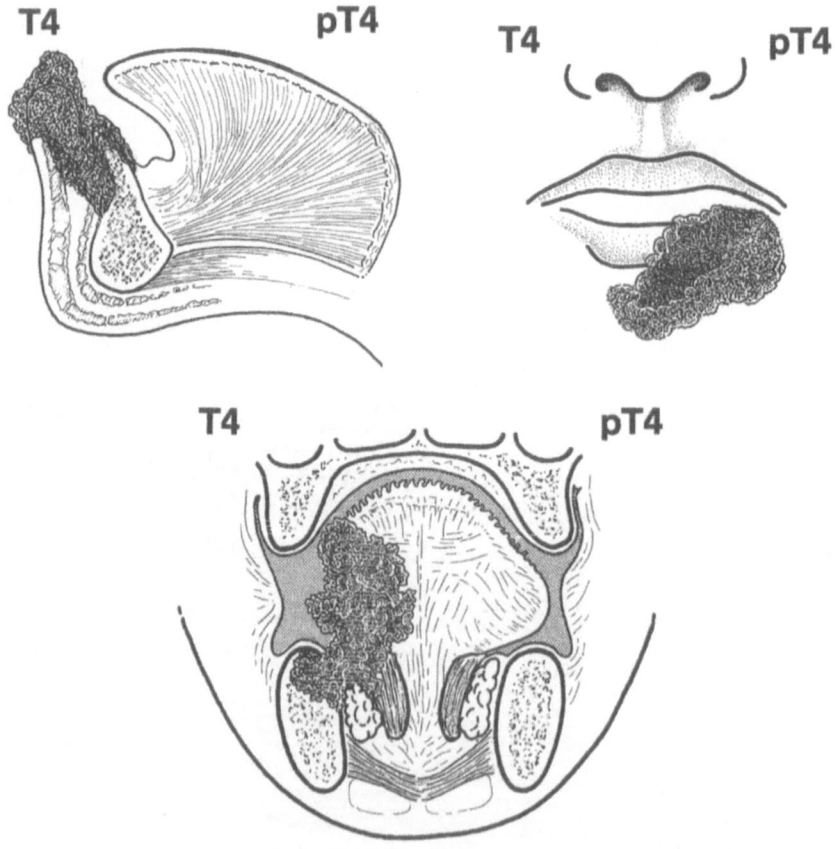

Regional Lymph Nodes

The regional lymph nodes are the cervical nodes. These include
(1) submental nodes
(2) submandibular nodes
(3) cranial jugular (deep cervical) nodes
(4) medial jugular (deep cervical) nodes
(5) caudal jugular (deep cervical) nodes
(6) dorsal cervical (superficial cervical) nodes along the accessory nerve
(7) supraclavicular nodes
(8) prelaryngeal and paratracheal nodes

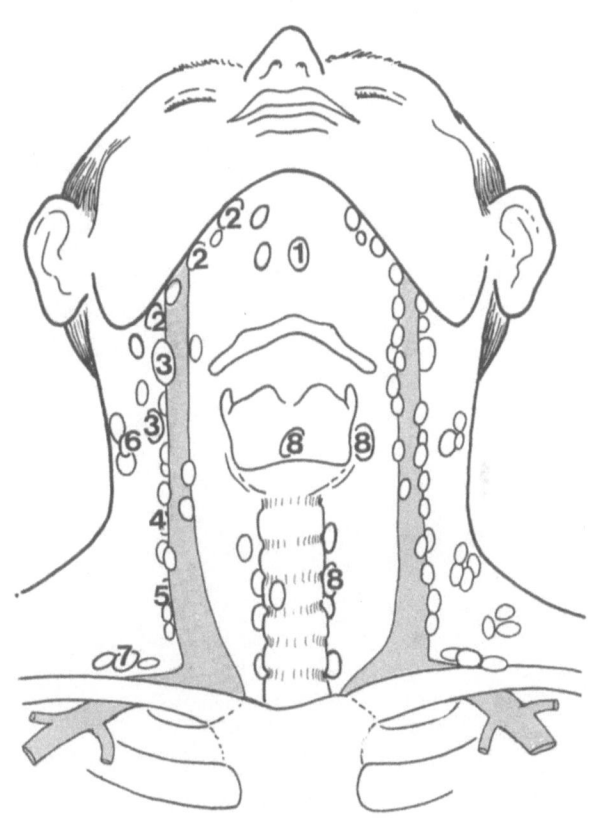

Regional Lymph Nodes (cont.)

 (9) retropharyngeal nodes
(10) parotid nodes
(11) buccal nodes
(12) retroauricular and occipital nodes

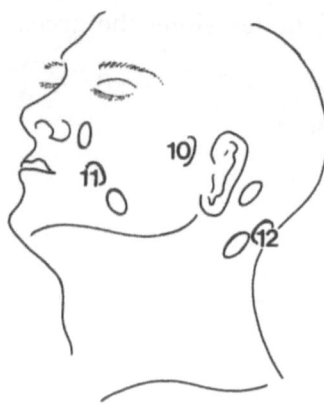
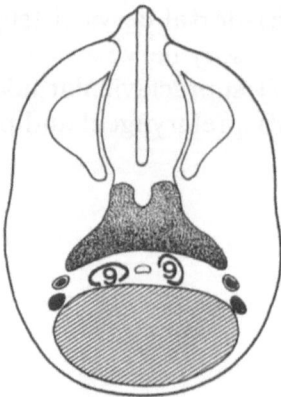

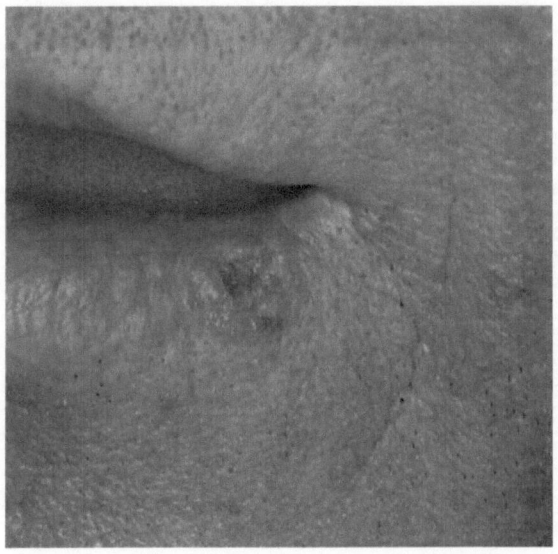

Fig. 1. *Cancer of the lower lip.* Ulcerated area surrounded by a firm, indurated margin

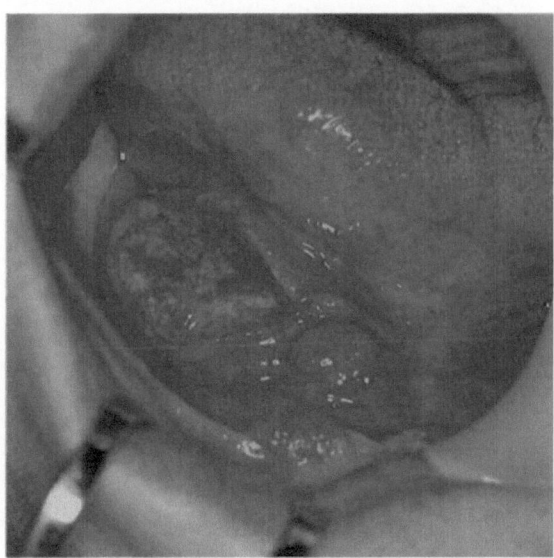

Fig. 2. *Cancer of the floor of the mouth.* Raw, ulcerated area with sharply defined margins

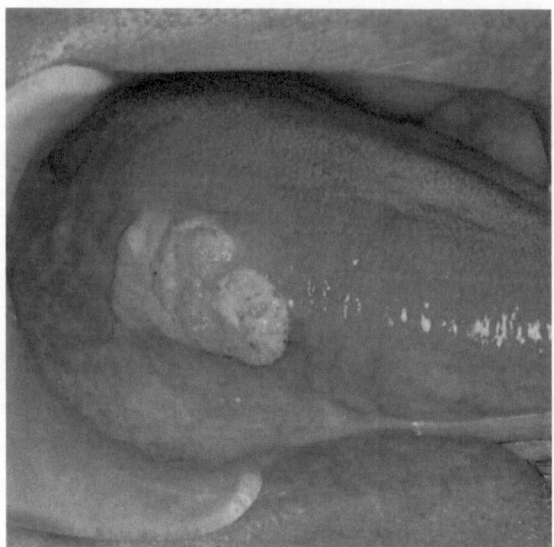

Fig. 3. *Cancer of lateral border of the tongue.* A predominantly white and warty growth

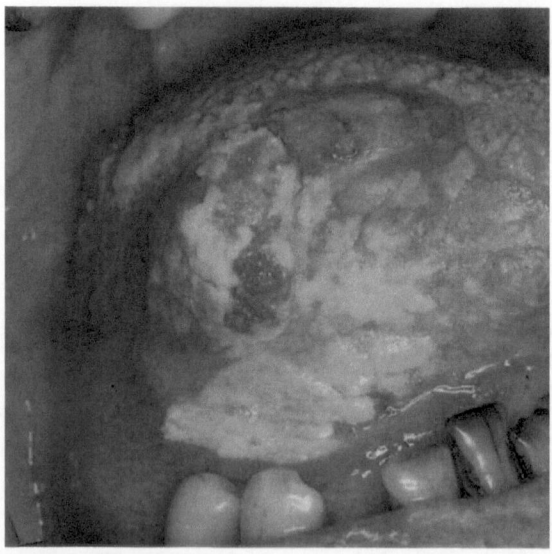

Fig. 4. *Cancer of lateral border of the tongue.* A raised red and white outgrowth surrounded by leukoplakia

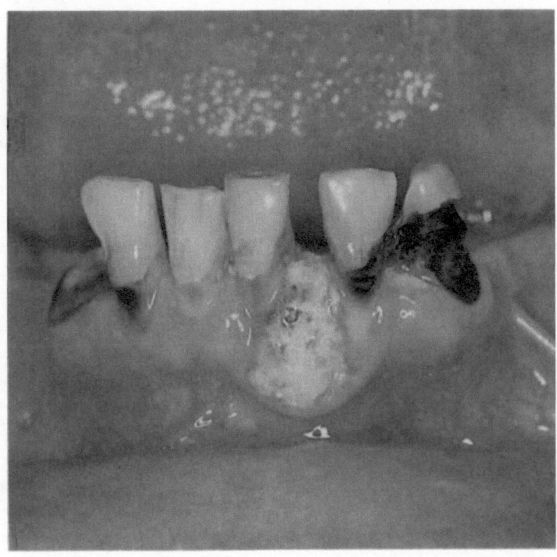

Fig. 5. *Cancer of mandibular gingiva*

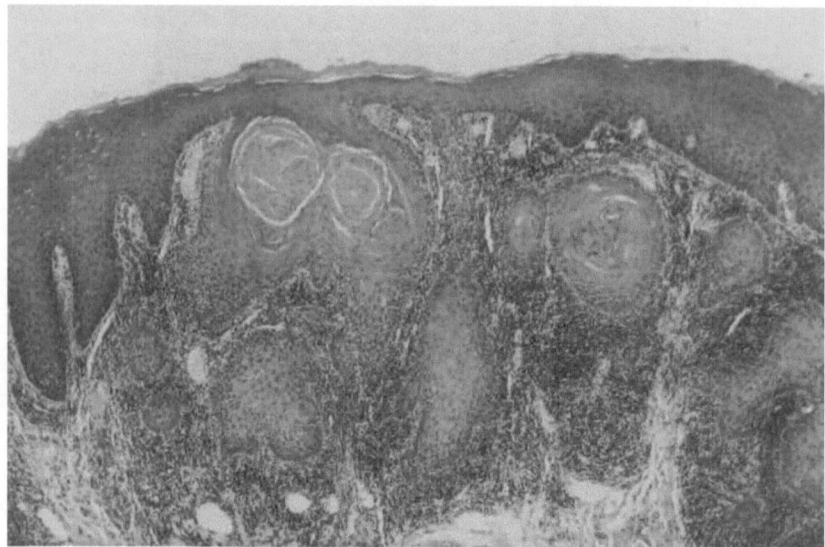

Fig. 6. *Squamous cell carcinoma, well differentiated.* Infiltrating nests and sheets of keratinizing squamous cell carcinoma

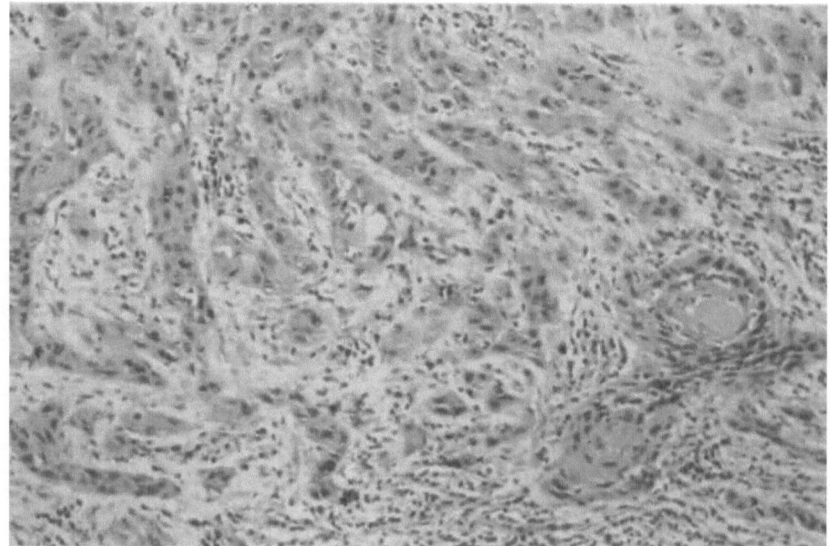

Fig. 7. *Squamous cell carcinoma, moderately differentiated.* Infiltrating islands and strands of squamous cell carcinoma with limited keratin formation

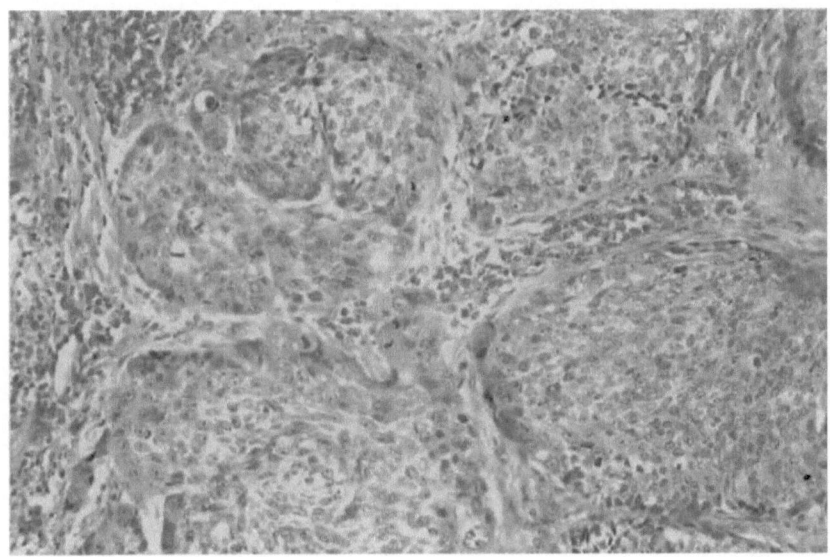

Fig. 8. *Squamous cell carcinoma, poorly differentiated.* Non-keratinizing sheets of infiltrating squamous cell carcinoma

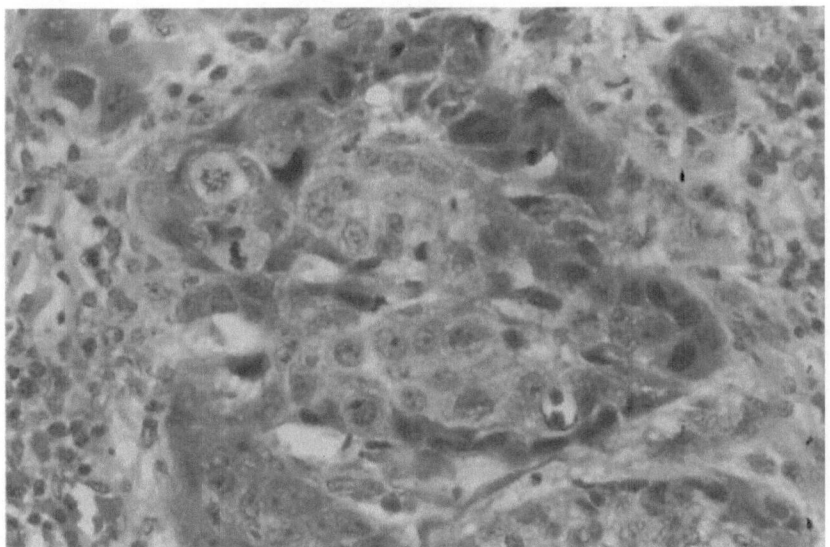

Fig. 9. *Squamous cell carcinoma, poorly differentiated.* Higher power view of part of same tumour as Fig. 8, showing wide variation in cellular and nuclear characteristics

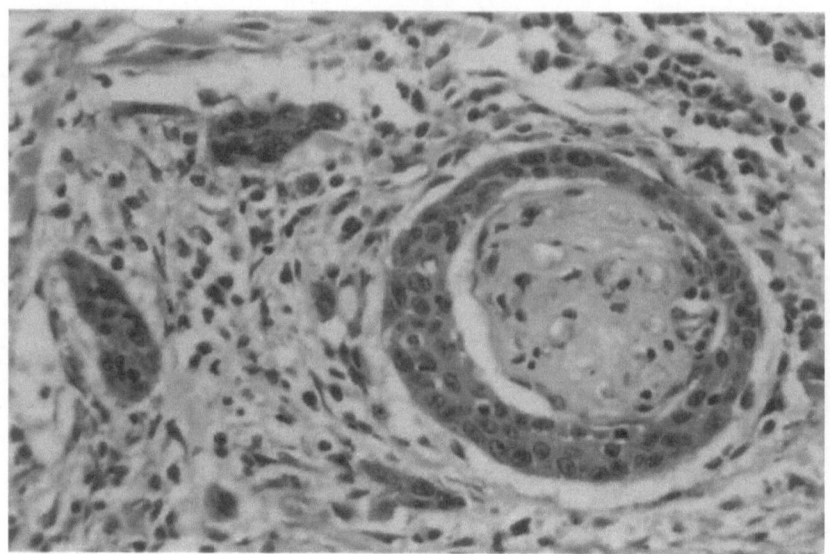

Fig. 10. *Squamous cell carcinoma*. Perineural infiltration

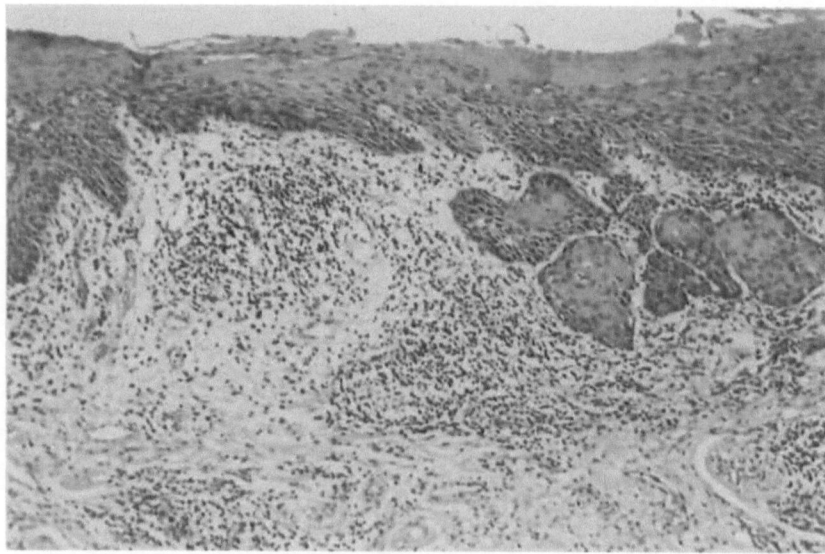

Fig. 11. *Squamous cell carcinoma, microinvasive type*. Shallow infiltration by islands of squamous cell carcinoma

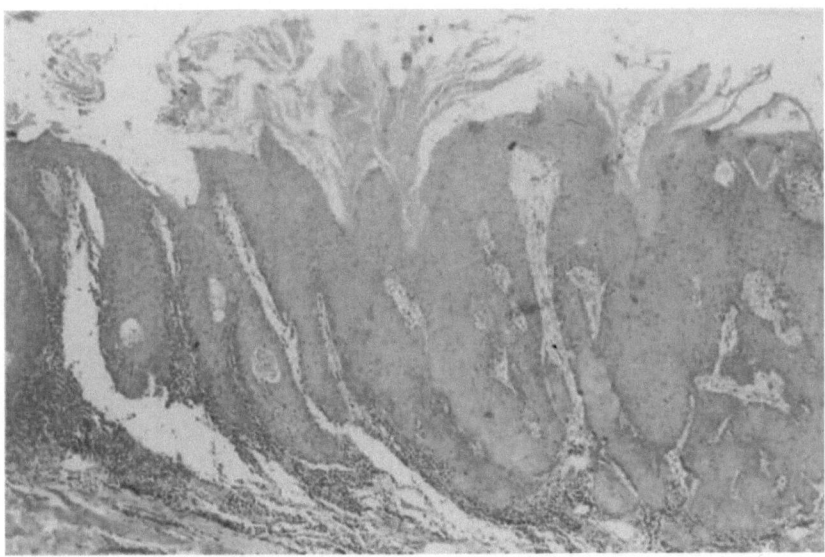

Fig. 12. *Papillary squamous cell carcinoma.* Squamous cell carcinoma composed mainly of exophytic papillary structures covered by hyperkeratinized epithelium

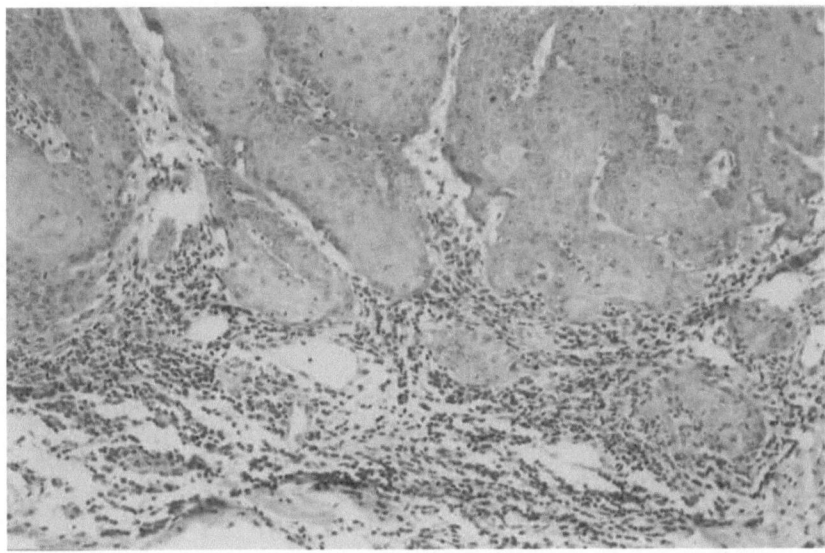

Fig. 13. *Papillary squamous cell carcinoma.* Part of same lesion as in Fig. 12 at higher magnification and showing infiltrating islands of squamous cell carcinoma

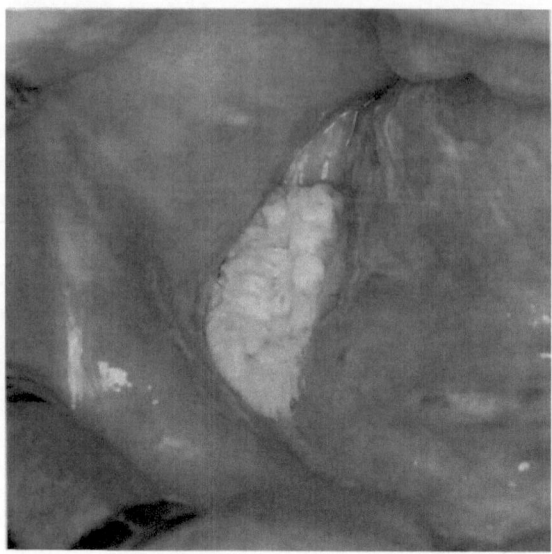

Fig. 14. *Verrucous carcinoma.* White papillary outgrowth on lower alveolar mucosa

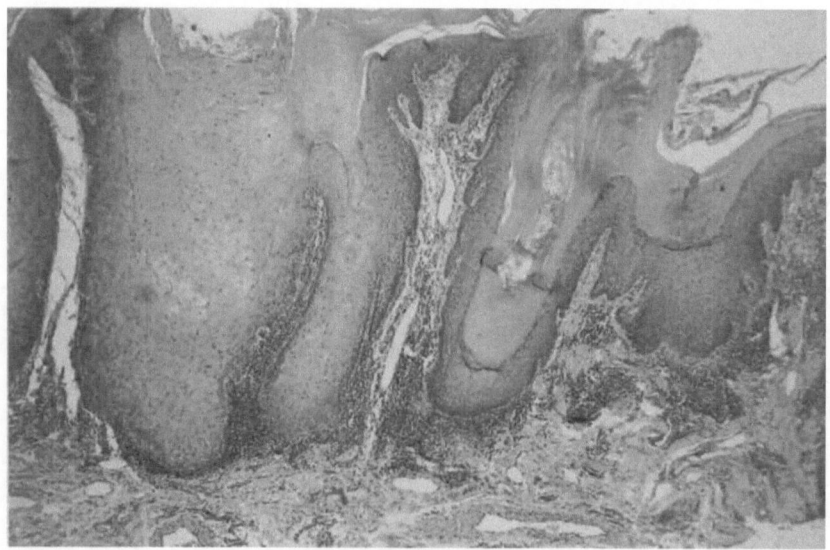

Fig. 15. *Verrucous carcinoma.* Exophytic hyperkeratinized papillary tumour with bland cytology and elongated epithelial rete-ridges

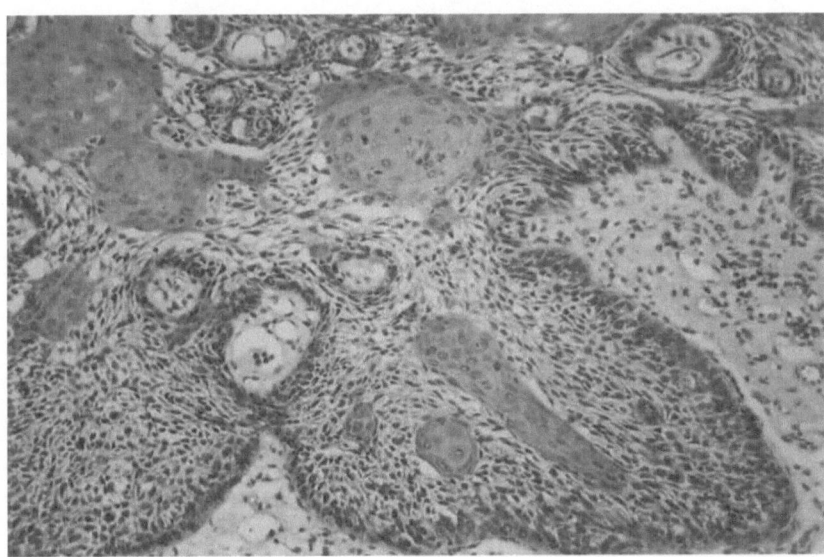

Fig. 16. *Basaloid squamous cell carcinoma.* Sheets of carcinoma cells with peripheral palisading and central focal squamous differentiation

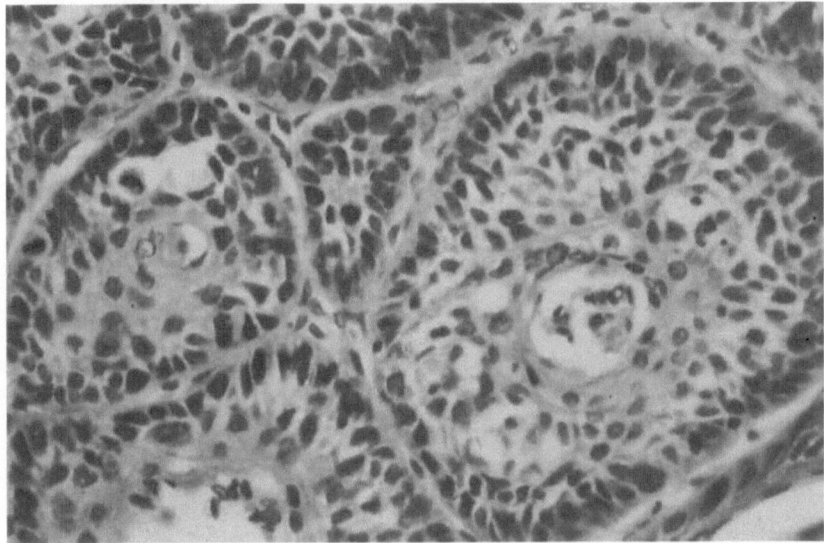

Fig. 17. *Basaloid squamous cell carcinoma.* Small cells with hyperchromatic nuclei show peripheral palisading and enclose areas of cystic necrosis

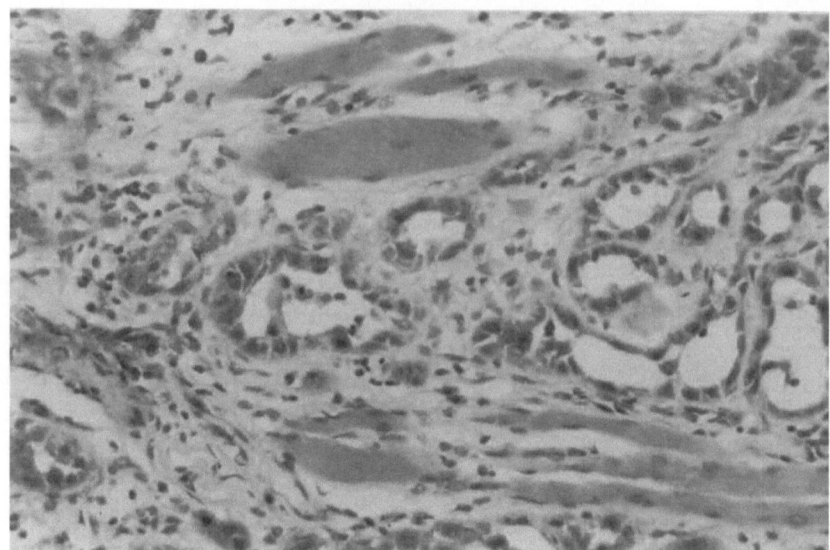

Fig. 18. *Adenoid squamous cell carcinoma.* Infiltrating islands of squamous cell carcinoma with acantholysis and pseudoglandular spaces

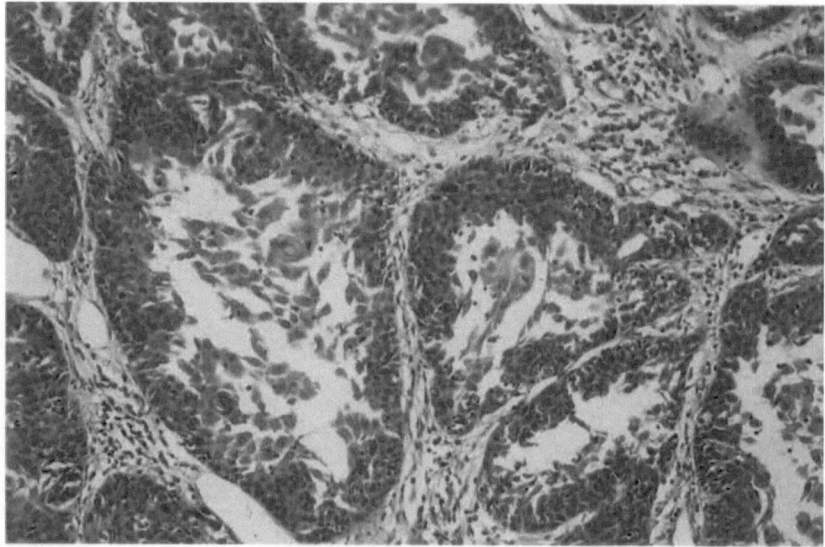

Fig. 19. *Adenoid squamous cell carcinoma*

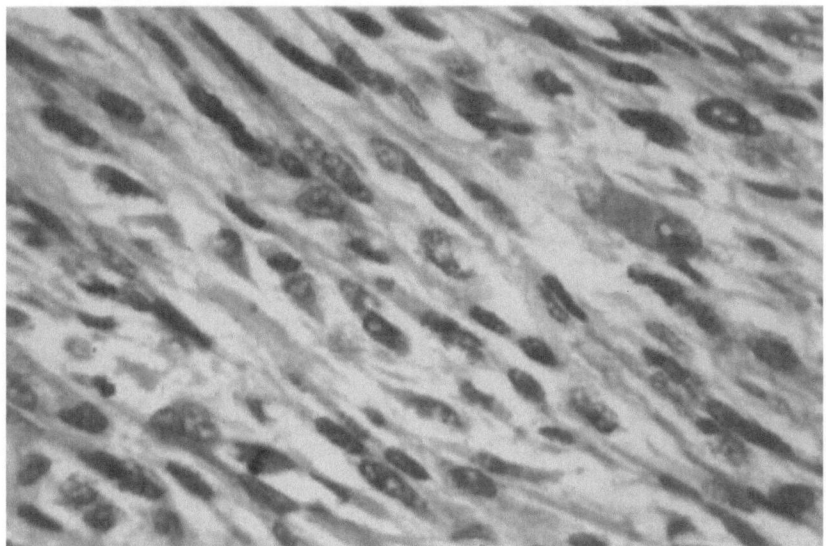

Fig. 20. *Spindle cell carcinoma*

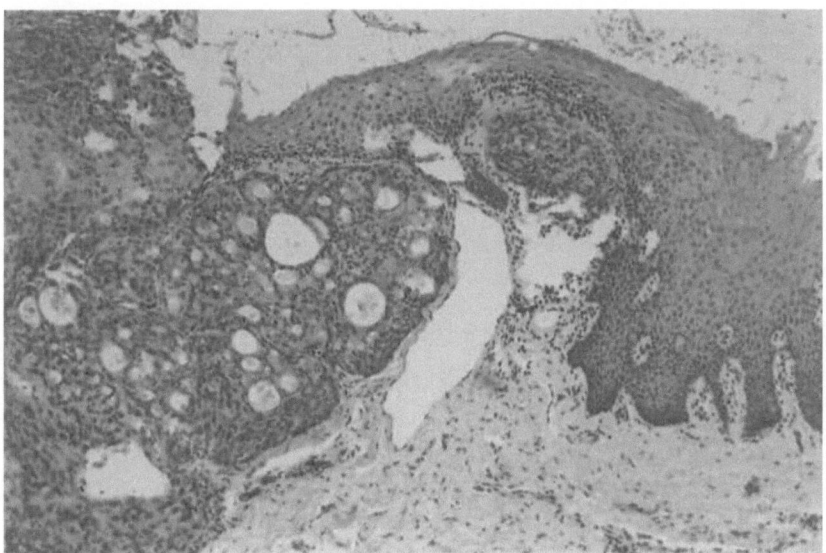

Fig. 21. *Adenosquamous carcinoma.* Infiltrating sheets of tumour cells with both adenocarcinoma and squamous cell carcinoma components

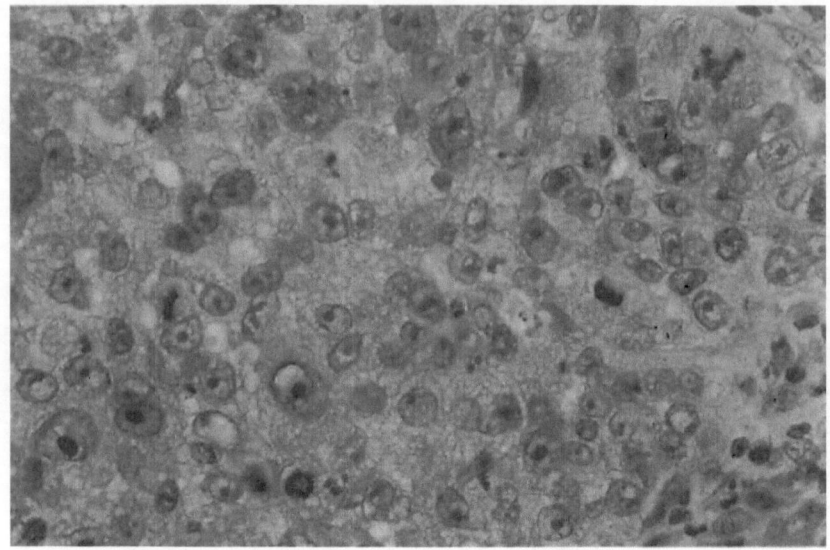

Fig. 22. *Undifferentiated carcinoma.* A syncytial mass of undifferentiated epithelial cells with vesicular nuclei and prominent nucleoli

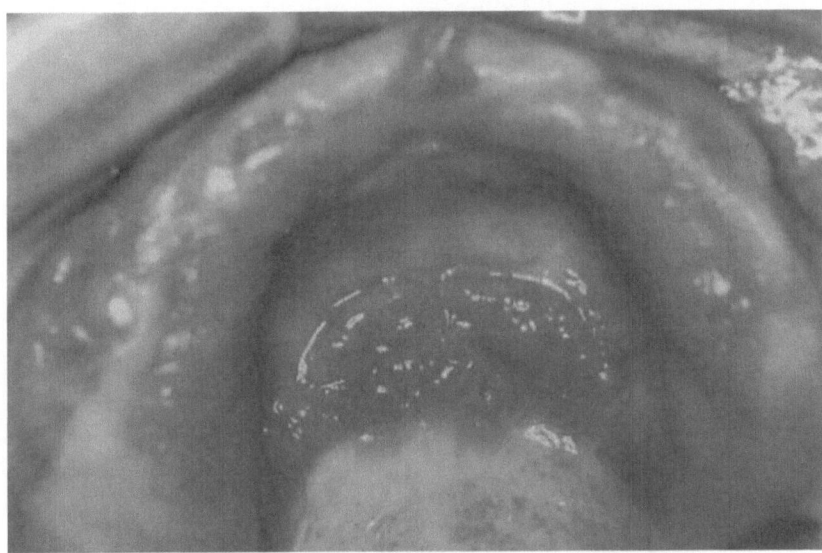

Fig. 23. *Papillary hyperplasia.* Red nodules on the hard palate mucosa

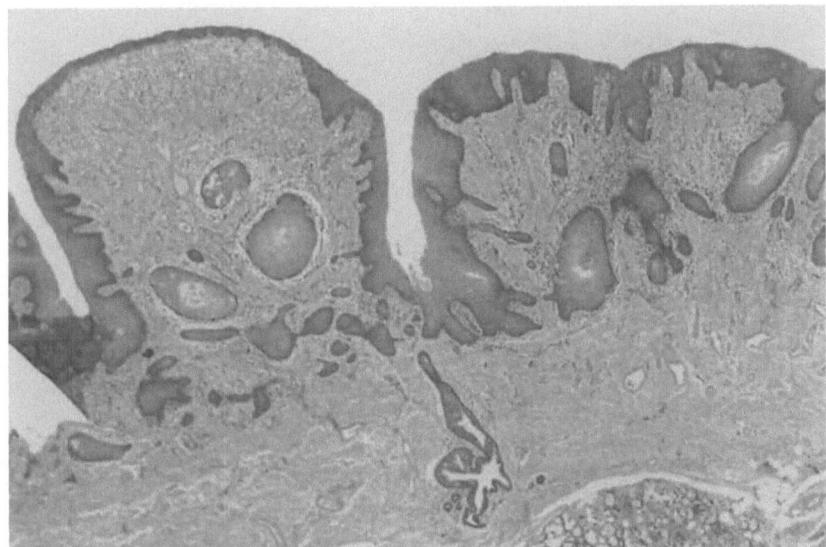

Fig. 24. *Papillary hyperplasia.* Hyperplastic and atrophic stratified squamous epithelium covers nodules of hyperplastic fibrous tissue; pseudoepitheliomatous hyperplasia is also evident

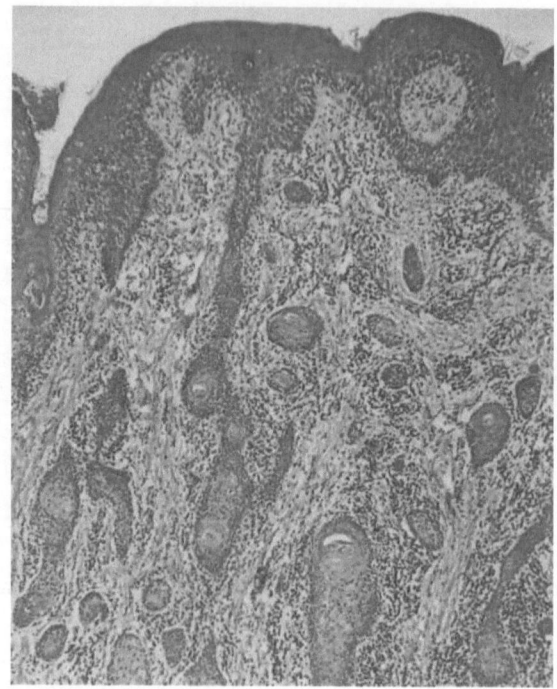

Fig. 25. *Papillary hyperplasia.* Florid pseudoepitheliomatous hyperplasia

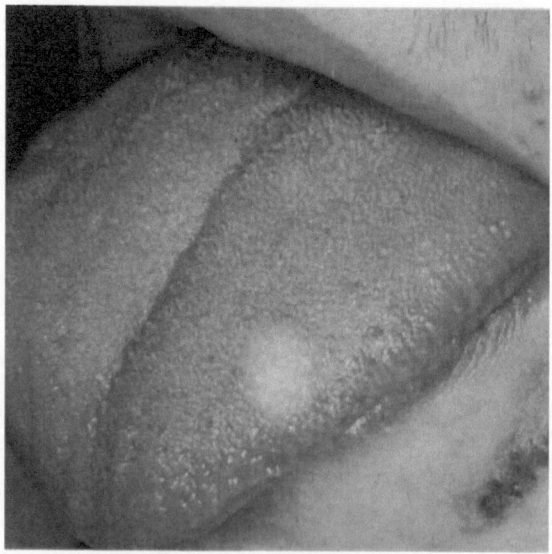

Fig. 26. *Granular cell tumour.* Raised white nodule on dorsum of tongue

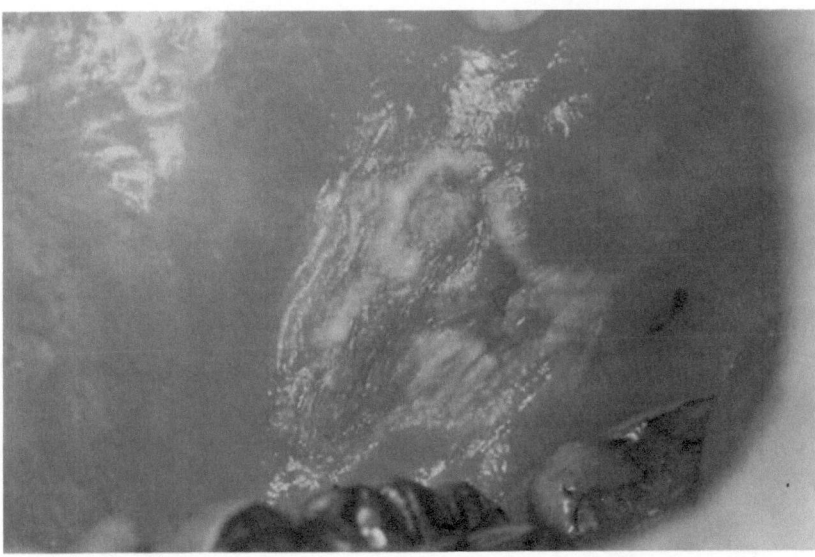

Fig.27. *Discoid lupus erythematosus.* Central red atrophic area on buccal mucosa surrounded by white mucosa showing some radiating striae

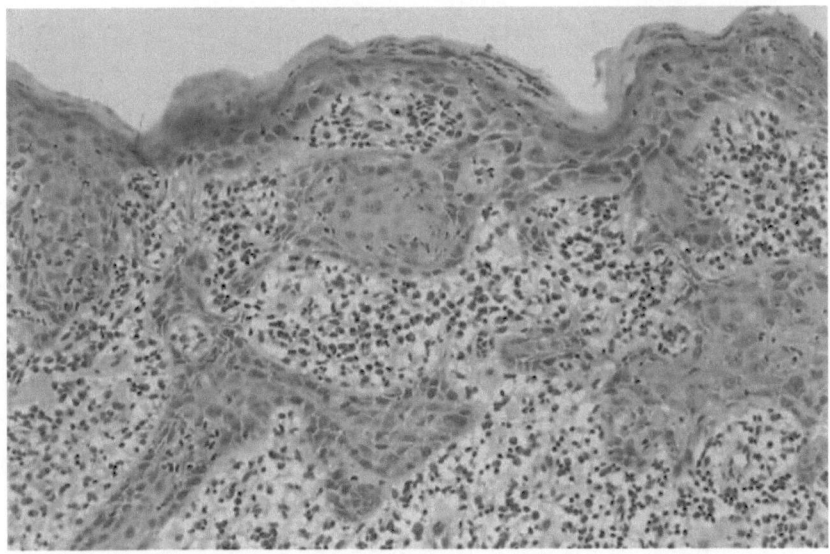

Fig.28. *Discoid lupus erythematosus.* Partly atrophic and hyperplastic stratified squamous epithelium is hyperkeratinized and exhibits pseudoepitheliomatous hyperplasia in a heavily inflamed stroma

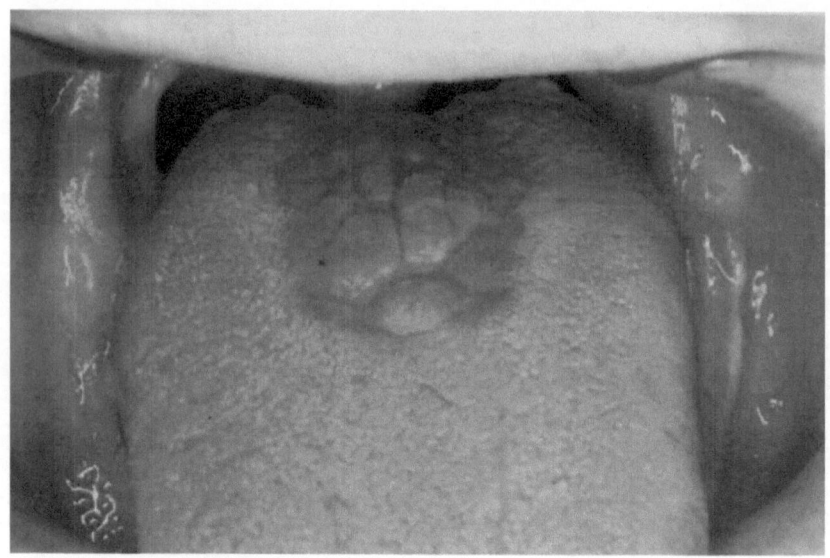

Fig. 29. *Median rhomboid glossitis.* Nodular de-papillated red area in midline of dorsum of tongue

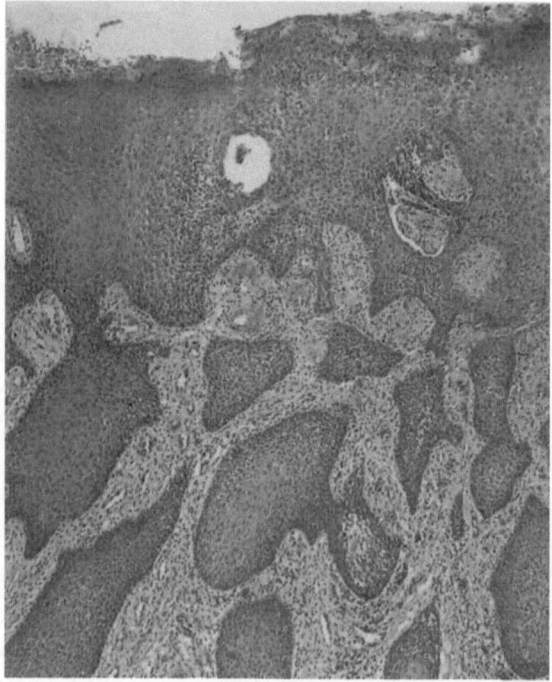

Fig. 30. *Median rhomboid glossitis.* Pseudoepitheliomatous hyperplasia

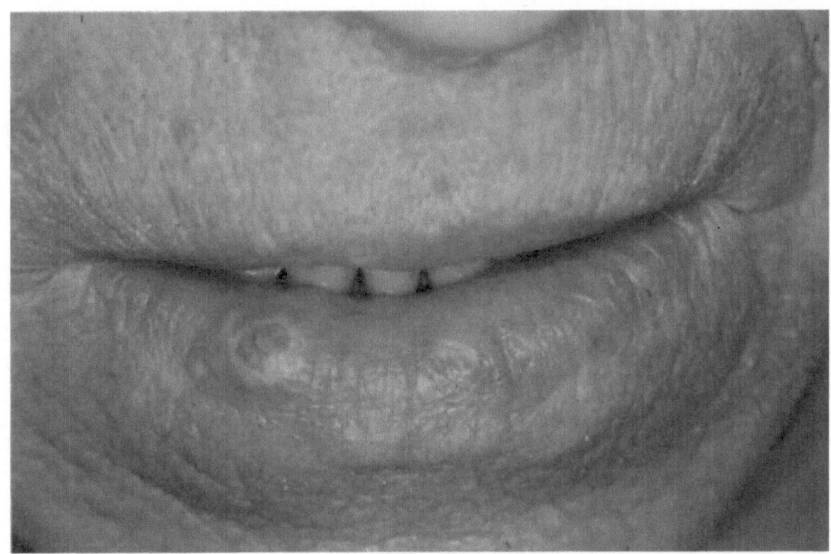

Fig. 31. *Keratoacanthoma of lower lip*

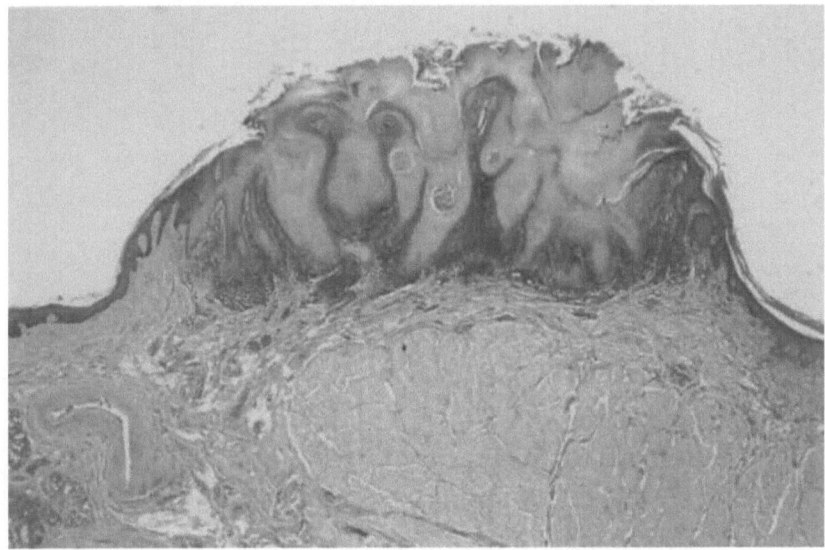

Fig. 32. *Keratoacanthoma*

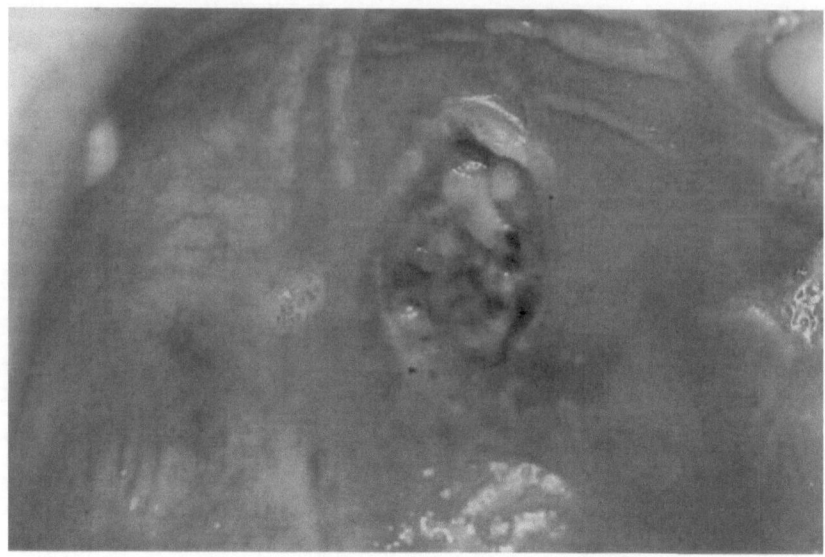

Fig. 33. *Necrotizing sialometaplasia.* Sharply defined necrotic ulcer on hard palate mucosa

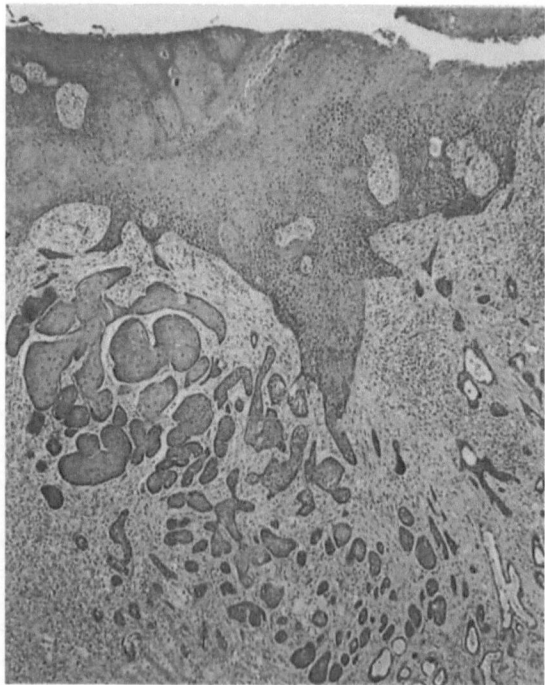

Fig. 34. *Necrotizing sialometaplasia.* Islands of metaplastic stratified squamous epithelium adjacent to necrotic tissue

59

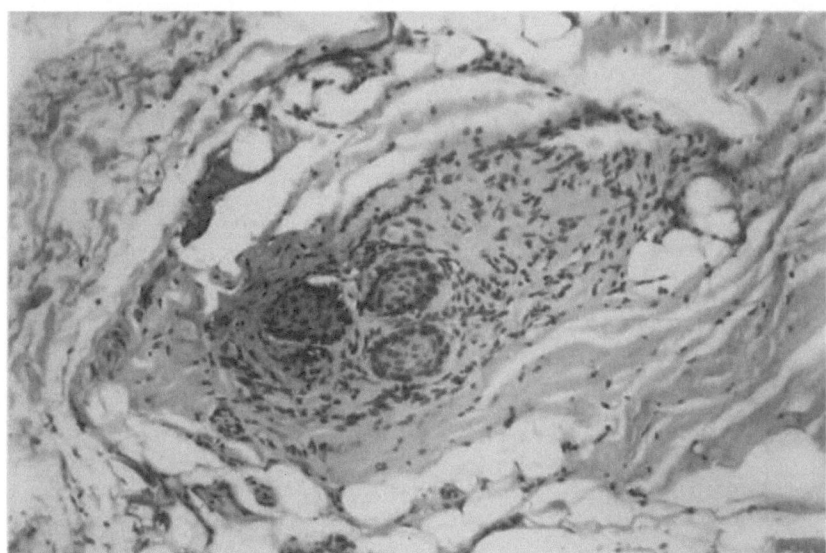

Fig.35. *Juxtaoral organ of Chievitz.* Islands of squamous epithelium among nerve fibres

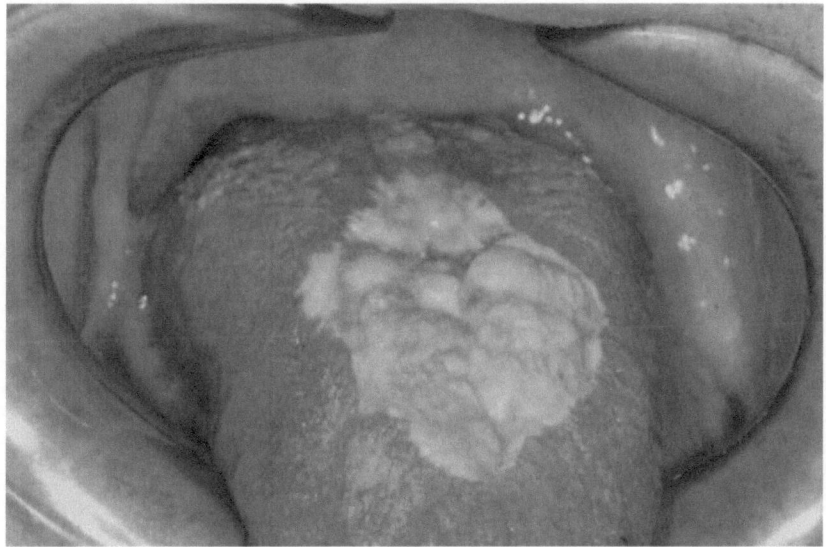

Fig.36. *Chronic hyperplastic candidiasis.* Nodular white and red plaque on dorsum of tongue

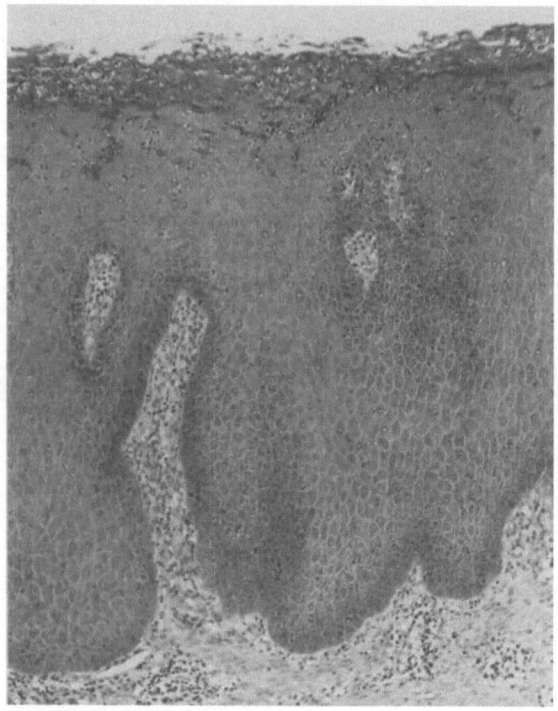

Fig. 37. *Chronic hyperplastic candidiasis.* Hyperplastic and atrophic parakeratinized stratified squamous epithelium

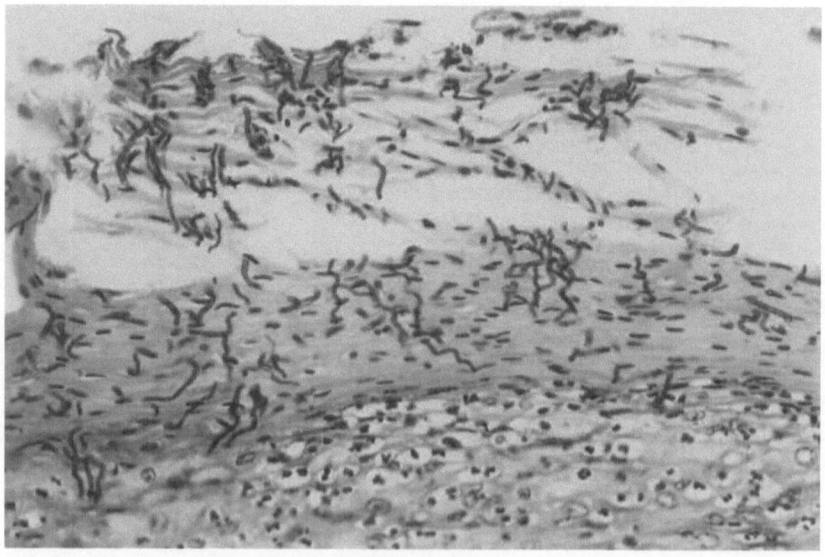

Fig. 38. *Chronic hyperplastic candidiasis.* Hyphae in parakeratinized zone. Periodic acid-Schiff stain

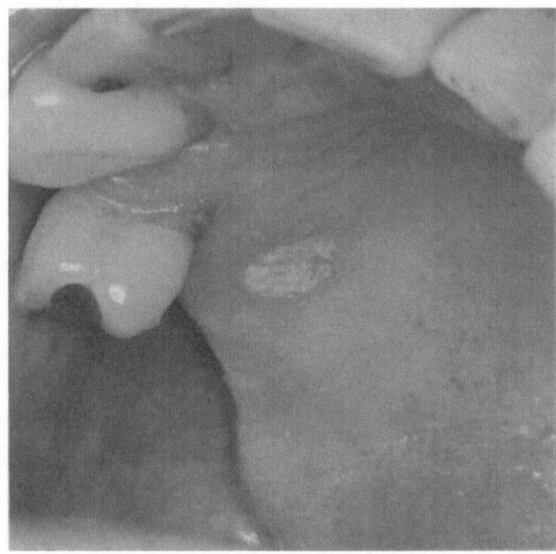

Fig. 39. *Verruciform xanthoma.* White sessile papillary lesion on palatal muco-sa

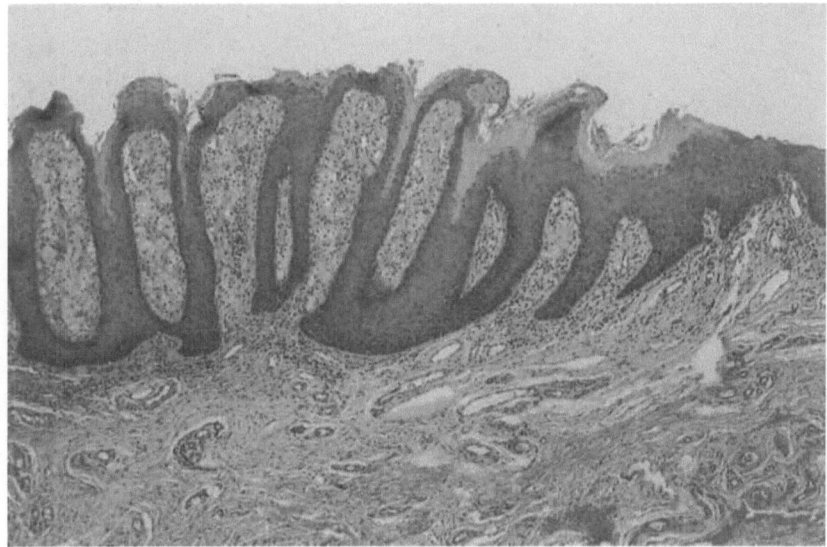

Fig. 40. *Verruciform xanthoma*

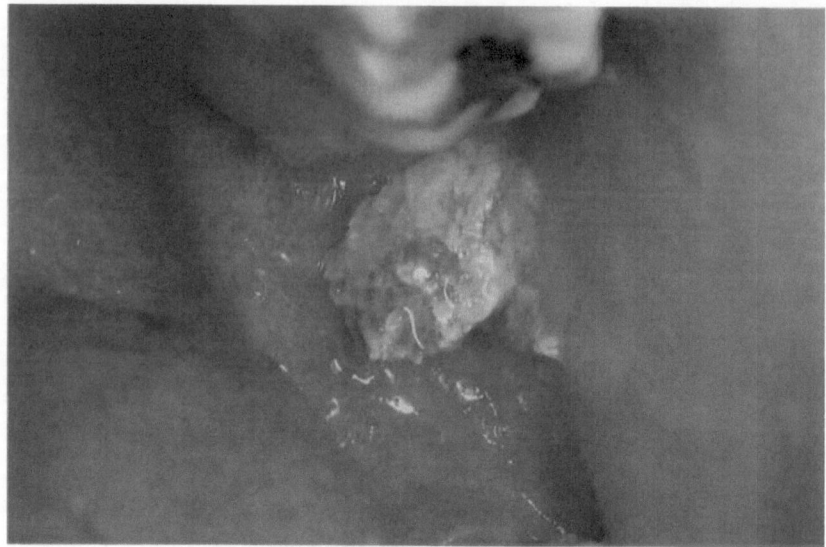

Fig. 41. *Verruca vulgaris.* Pedunculated pink papillary mass on posterior aspect of buccal mucosa

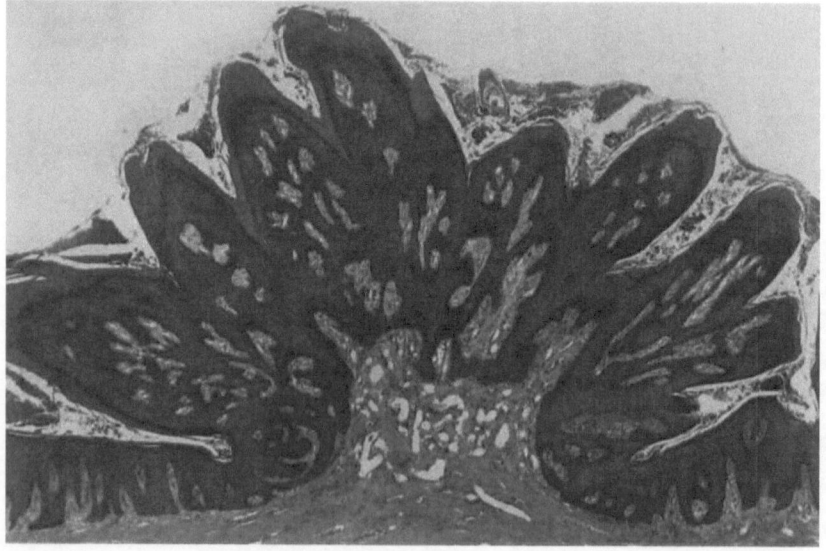

Fig. 42. *Verruca vulgaris*

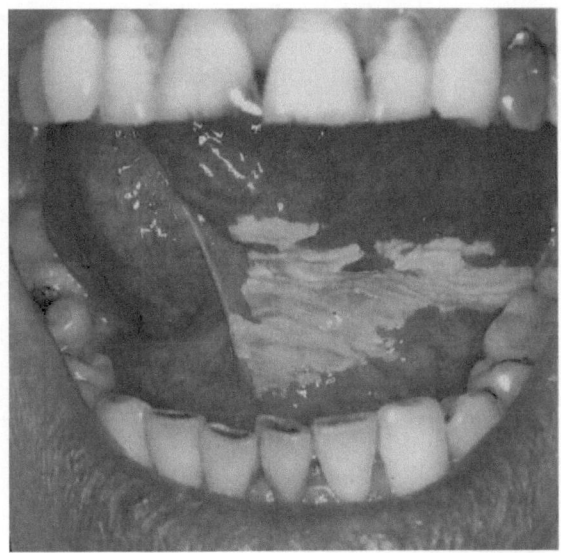

Fig. 43. *Homogeneous leukoplakia, floor of mouth mucosa.* Corrugated type

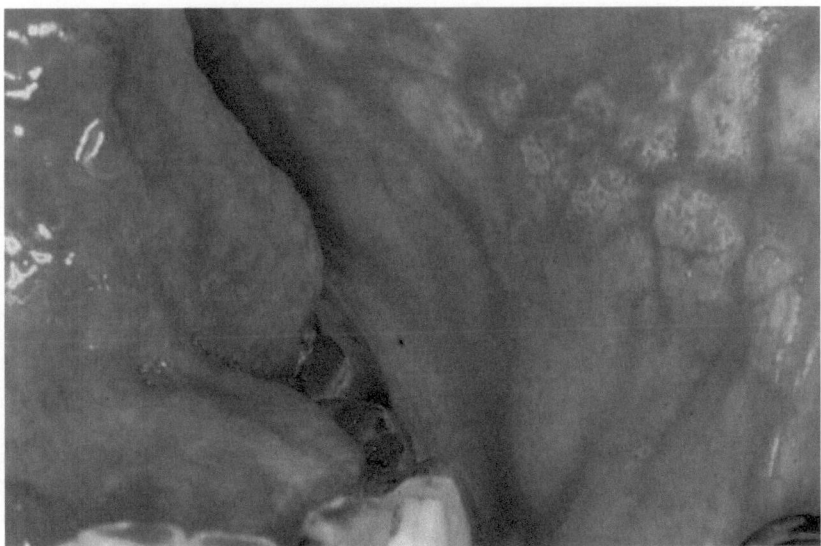

Fig. 44. *Homogeneous leukoplakia, buccal mucosa.* Pumice-like type

64

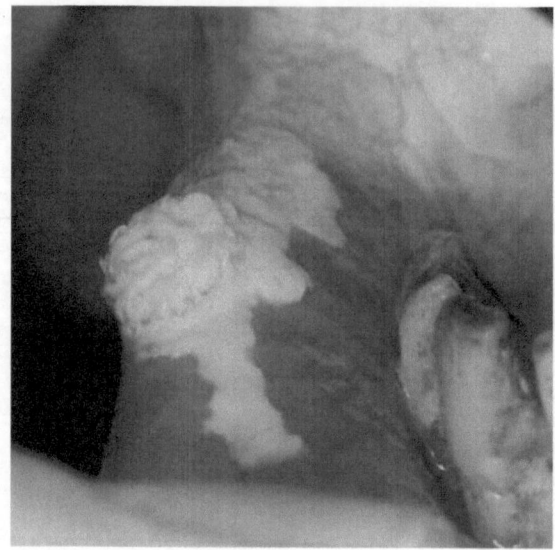

Fig. 45. *Non-homogeneous leukoplakia, labial mucosa.* Verrucous type

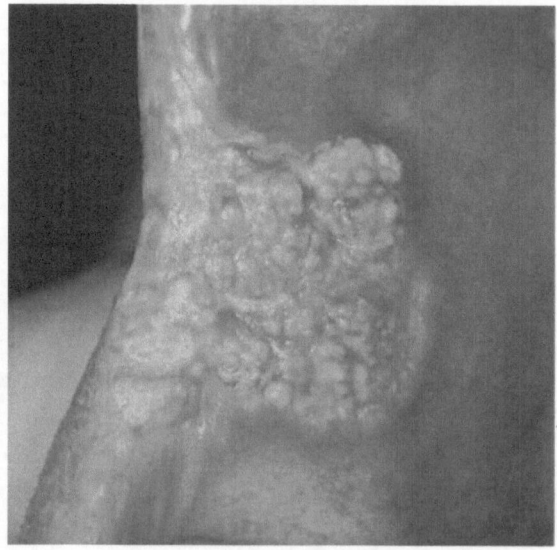

Fig. 46. *Non-homogeneous leukoplakia, commissure region.* Nodular type

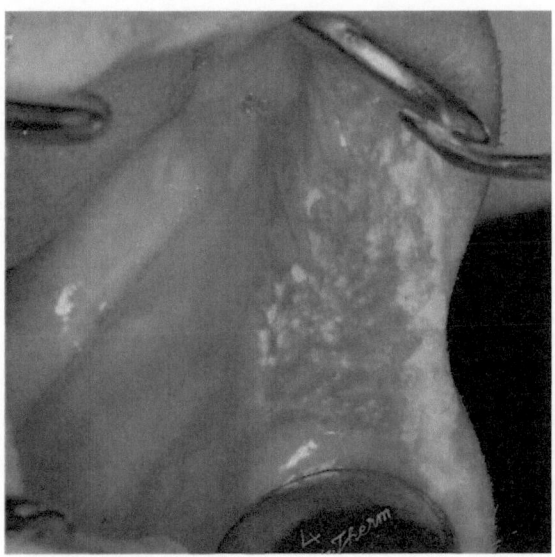

Fig. 47. *Erythroleukoplakia of commissure region*

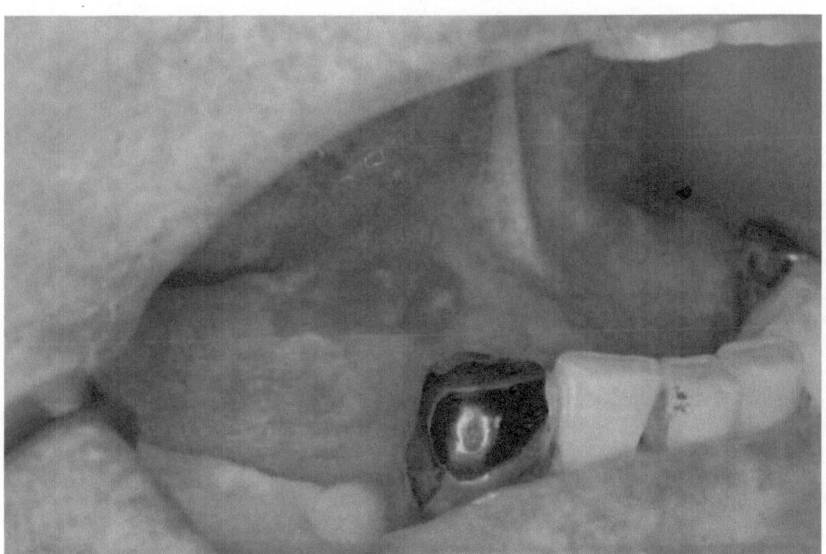

Fig. 48. *Erythroplakia, floor of mouth mucosa*

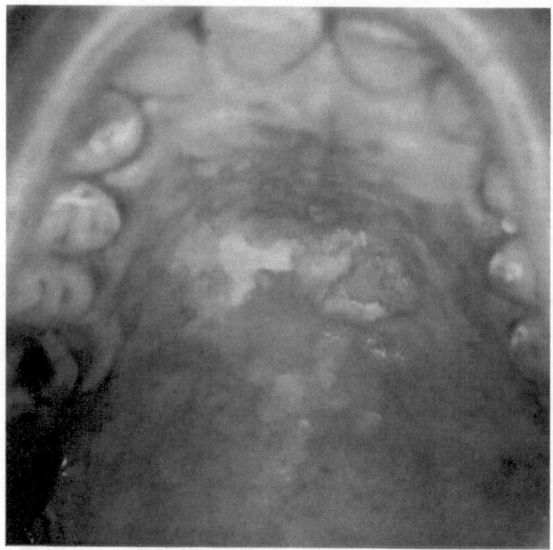

Fig. 49. *Palatal keratosis in a reverse smoker*

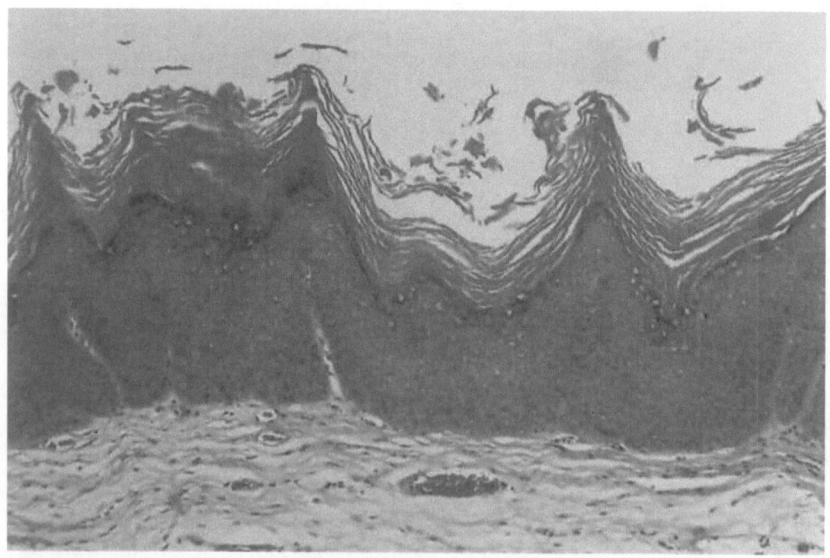

Fig. 50. *Hyperorthokeratosis without epithelial dysplasia*

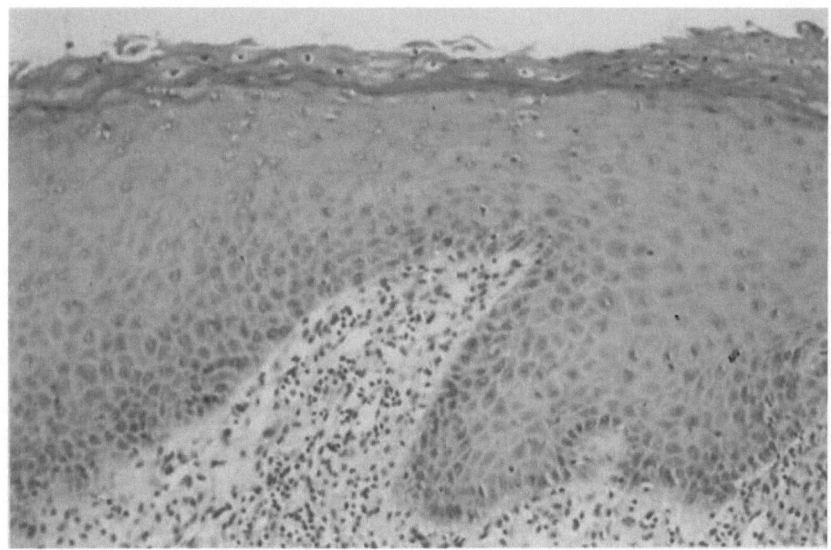

Fig. 51. *Hyperparakeratosis without epithelial dysplasia*

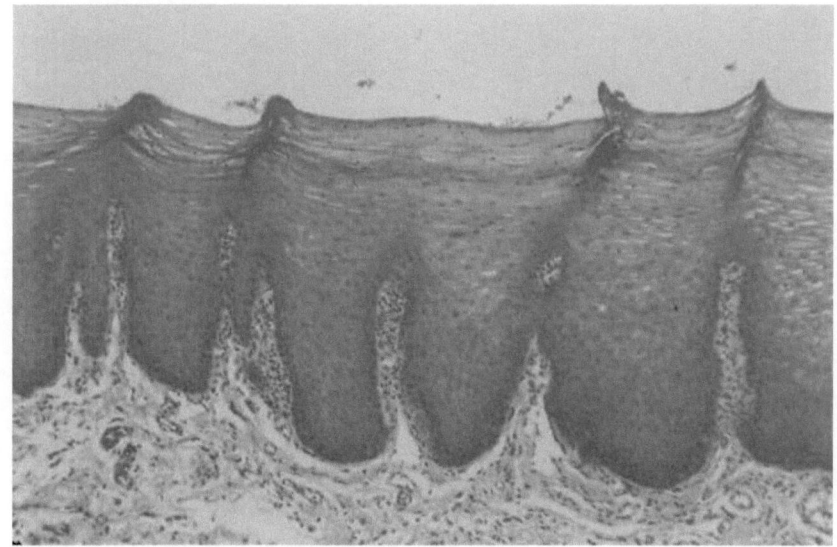

Fig. 52. *Chevron-type keratinization*

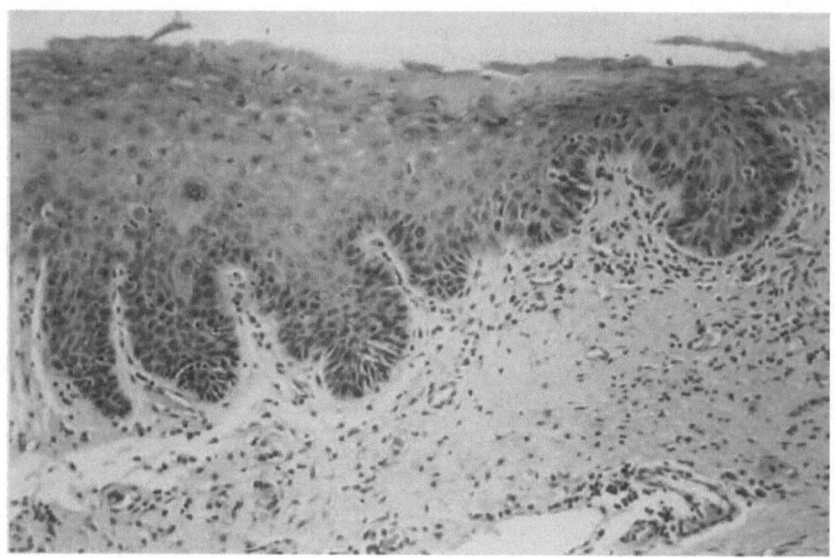

Fig. 53. *Mild squamous epithelial dysplasia*

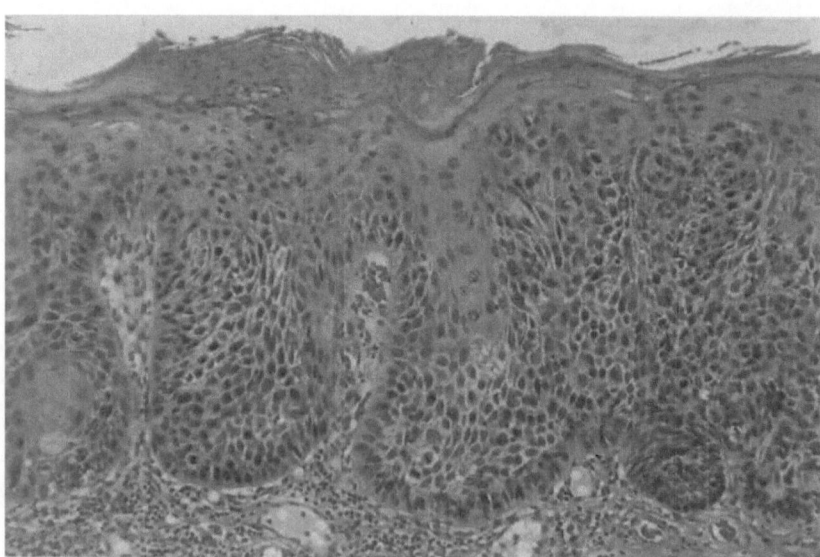

Fig. 54. *Moderate squamous epithelial dysplasia*

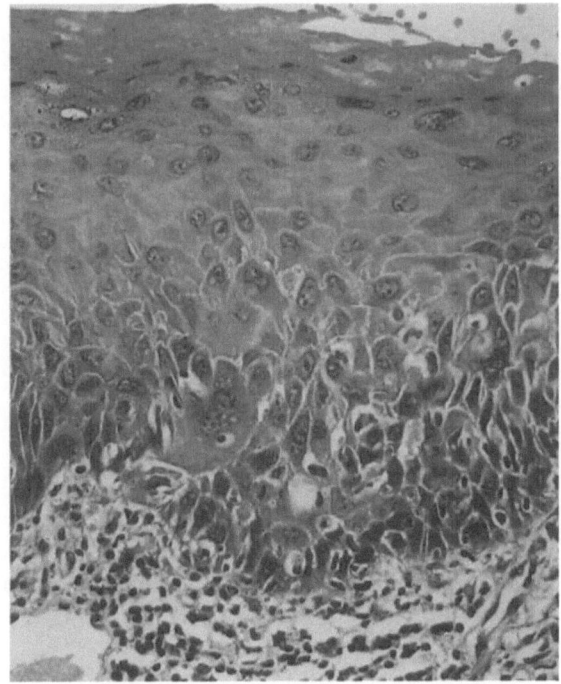

Fig.55. *Severe squamous epithelial dysplasia*

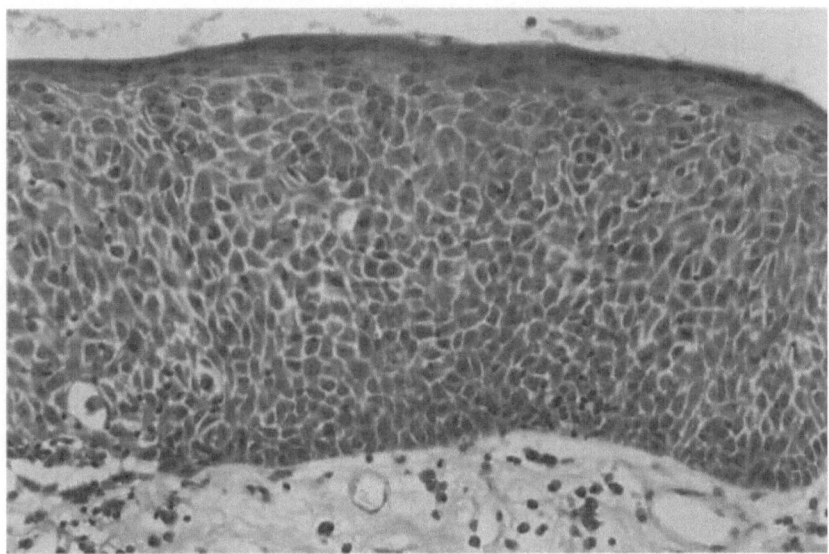

Fig.56. *Squamous cell carcinoma in situ*

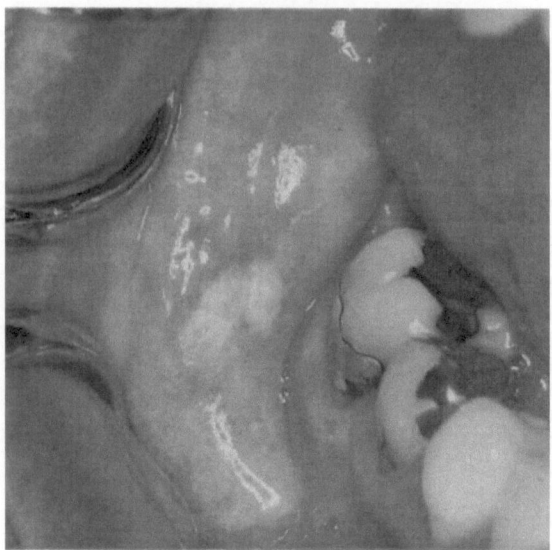

Fig. 57. *White lesion on buccal mucosa in contact with an amalgam restoration*

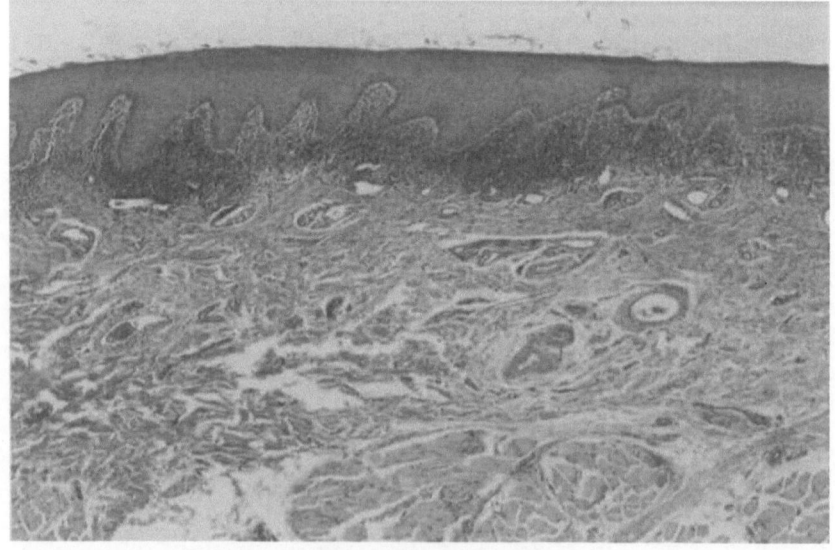

Fig. 58. *Lichenoid changes in lesion shown in Fig. 57*

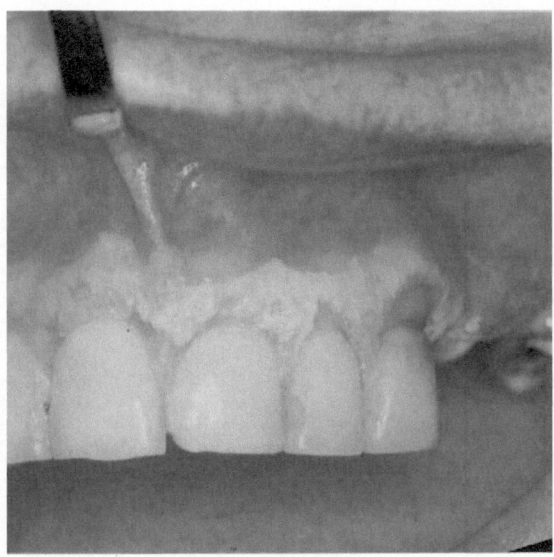

Fig. 59. *Frictional keratosis of gingival mucosa*

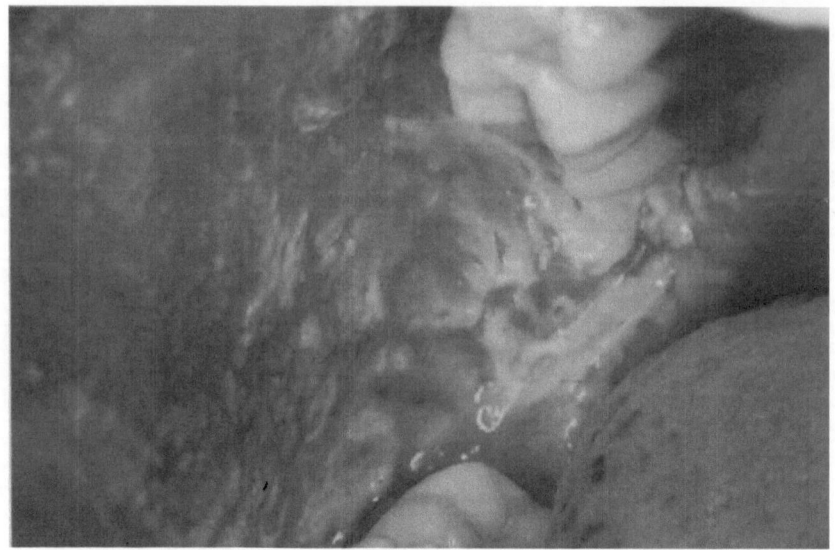

Fig. 60. *White sponge naevus, buccal mucosa*

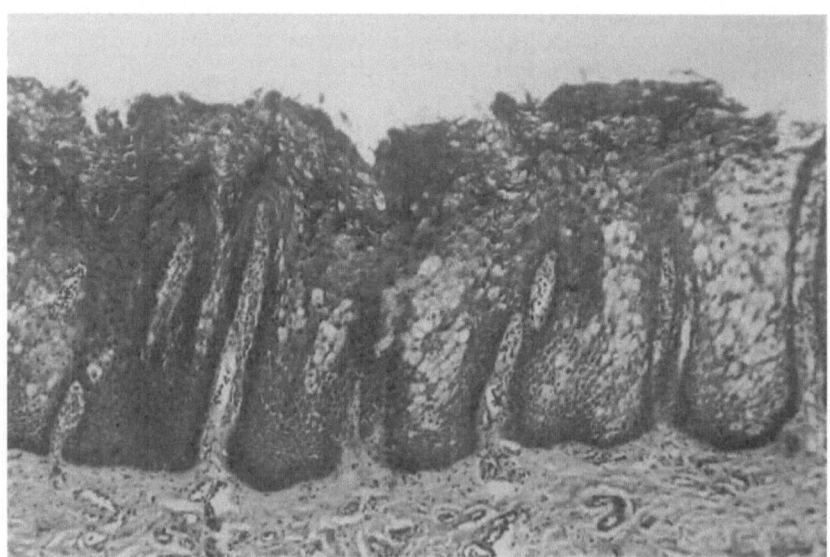

Fig. 61. *White sponge naevus*

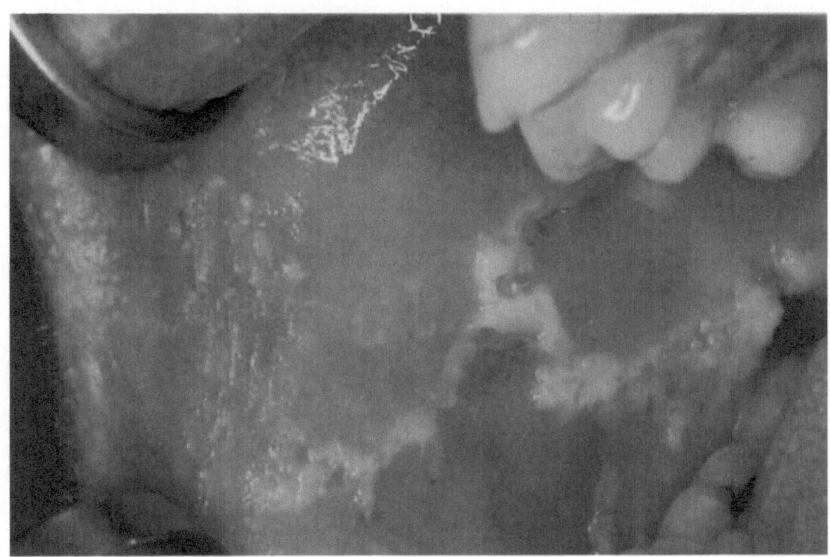

Fig. 62. *Cheek-biting (morsicatio buccarum)*

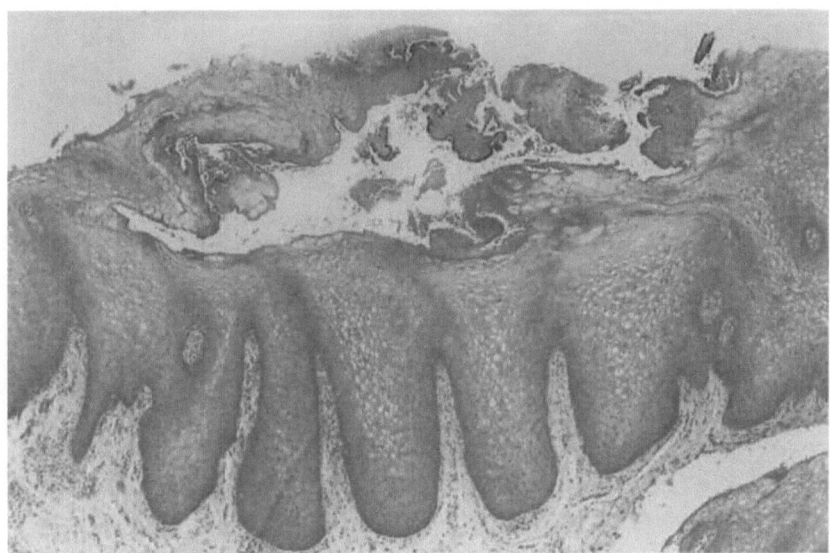

Fig. 63. *Cheek-biting*

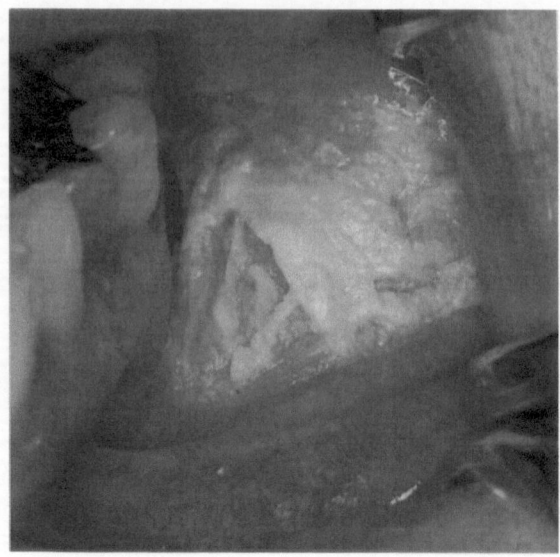

Fig. 64. *Aspirin burn, buccal mucosa*

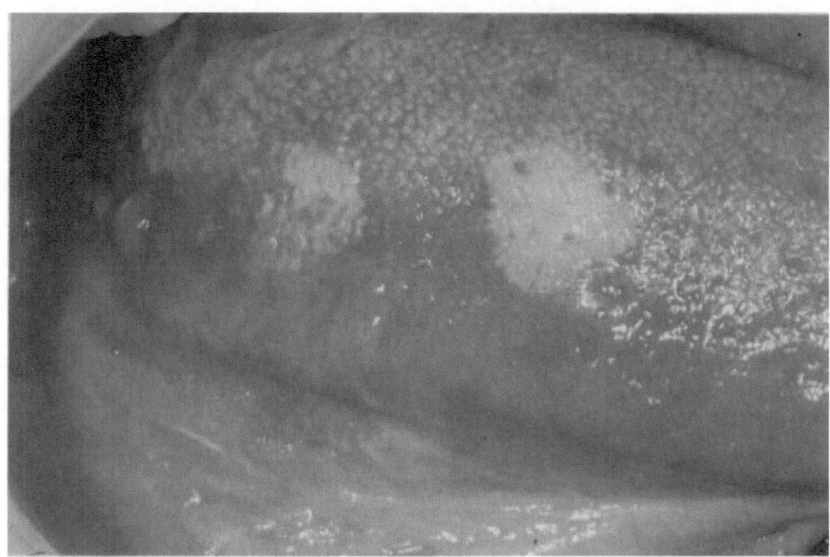

Fig. 65. *Lichen planus, lateral border of tongue.* Plaque-like type

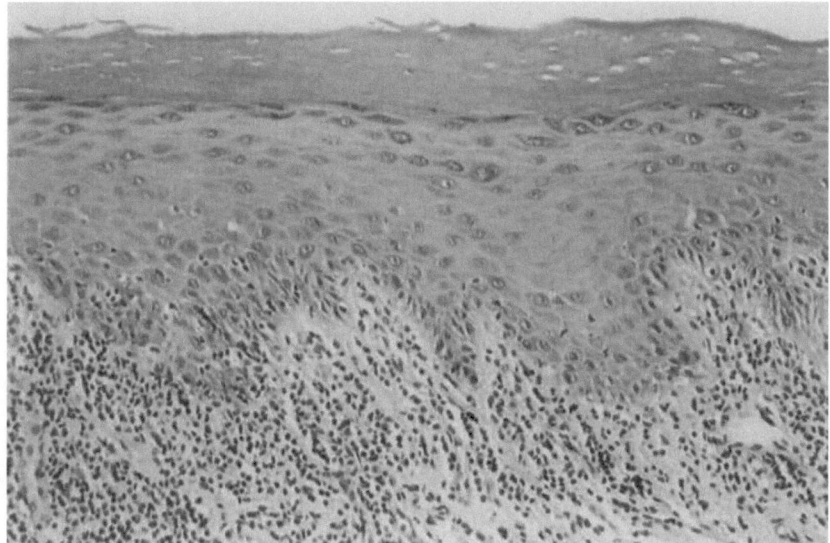

Fig. 66. *Lichen planus*

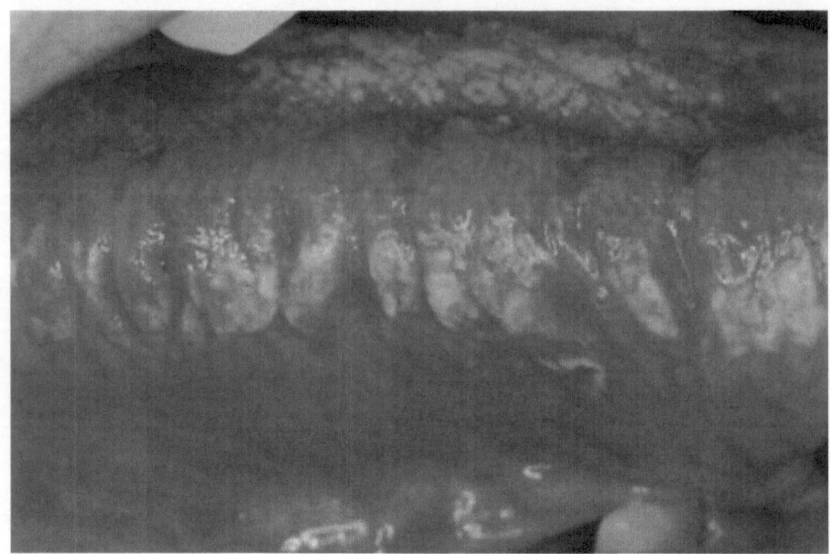

Fig. 67. *Hairy leukoplakia, lateral border of tongue*

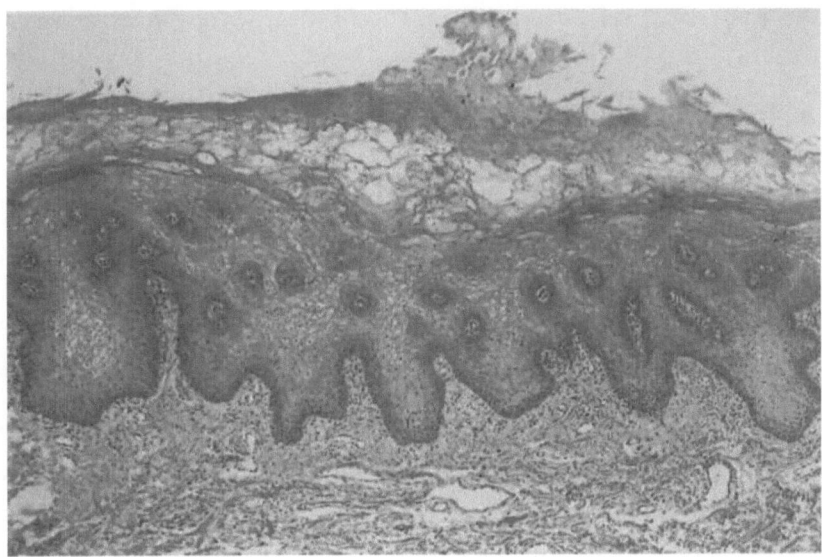

Fig.68. *Hairy leukoplakia*

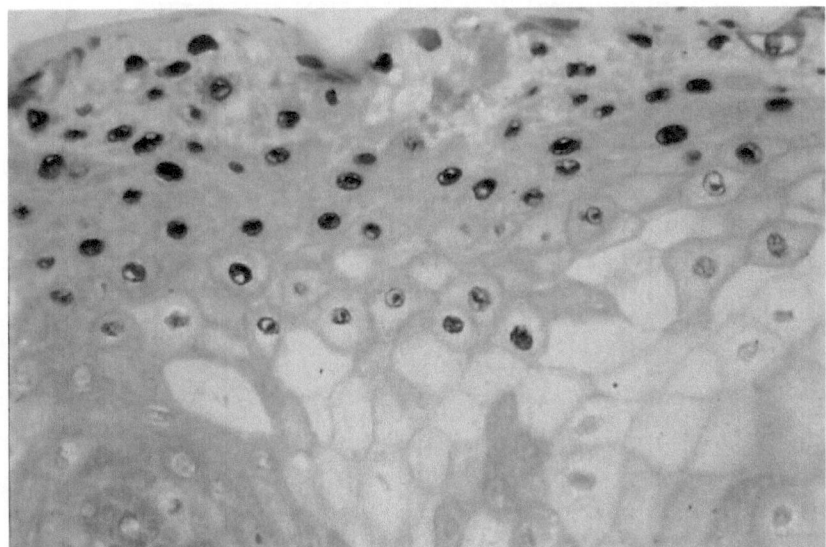

Fig.69. *Hairy leukoplakia.* Epstein–Barr virus (EBV) DNA-positive in superficial epithelial cell nuclei by in situ hybridization

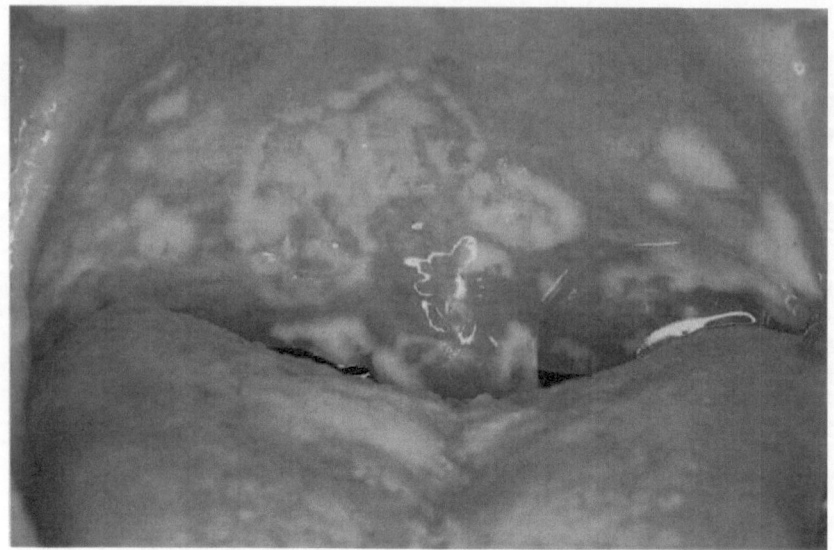

Fig. 70. *Pseudomembranous candidiasis (thrush), soft palate mucosa*

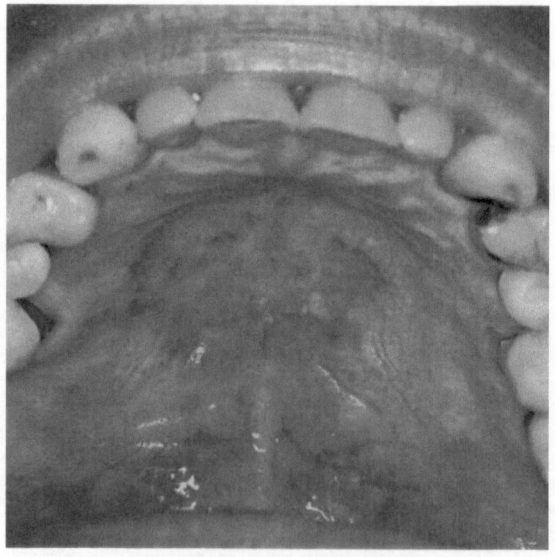

Fig. 71. *Erythematous candidiasis, hard palate mucosa*

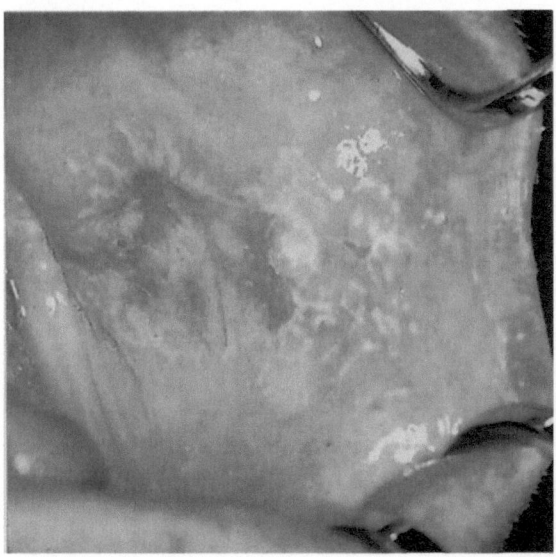

Fig. 72. *Erosive lichen planus, buccal mucosa.* Red areas surrounded by striated white mucosa

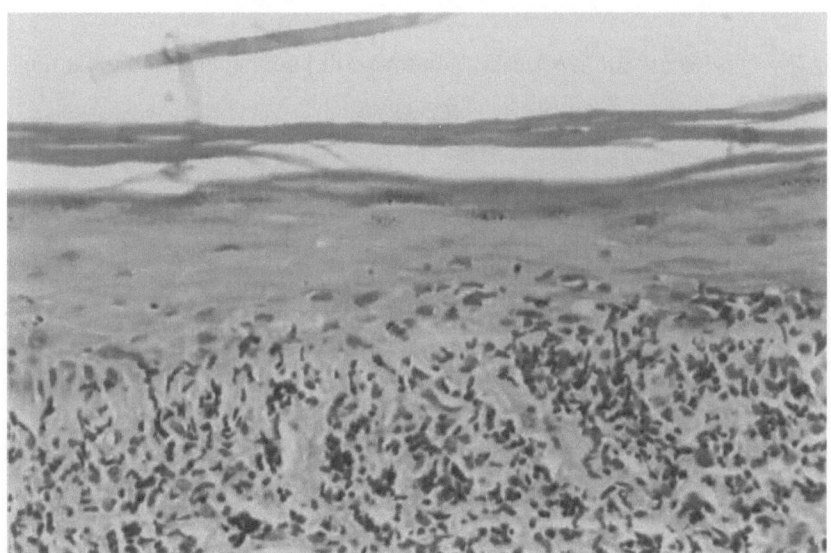

Fig. 73. *Erosive lichen planus*

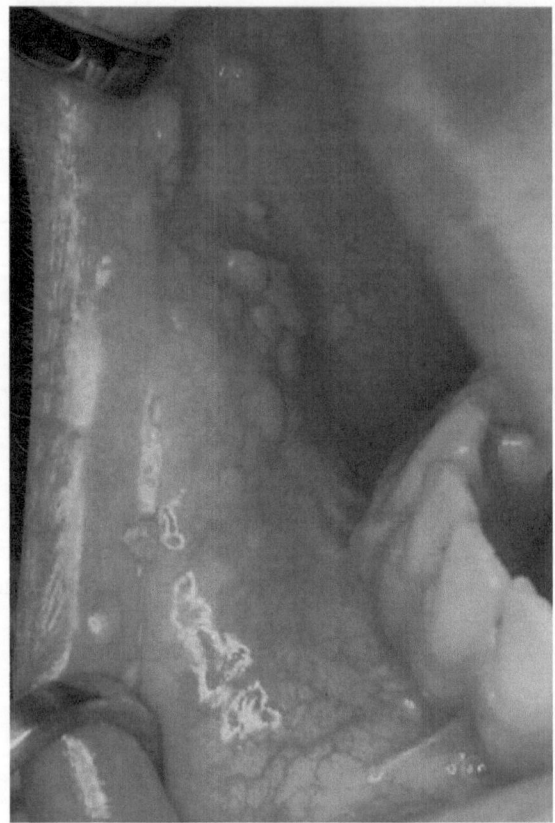

Fig. 74. *Focal epithelial hyperplasia.* Multiple soft pink papules on buccal mucosa

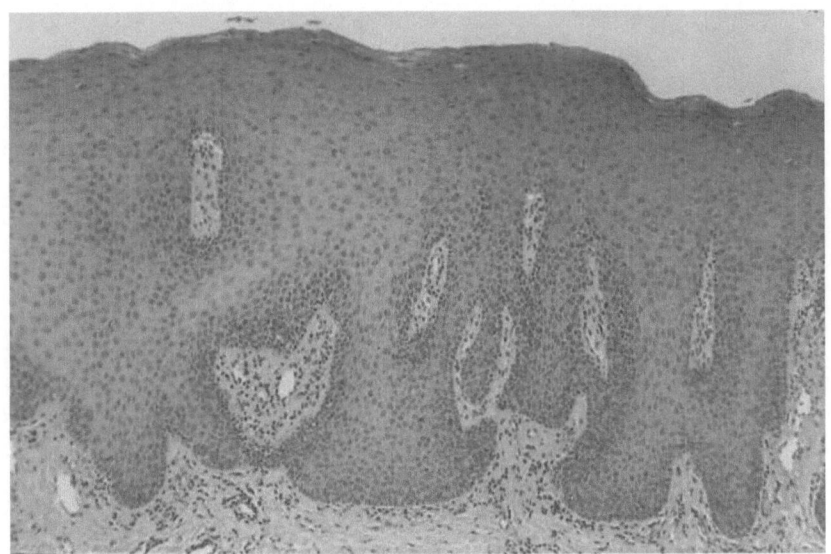

Fig. 75. *Focal epithelial hyperplasia*

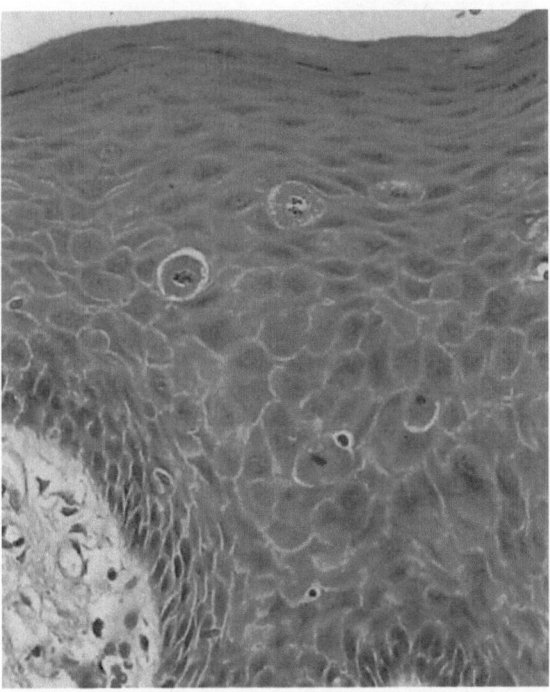

Fig. 76. *Focal epithelial hyperplasia.* Mitosoid cells in spinous layer of stratified squamous epithelium

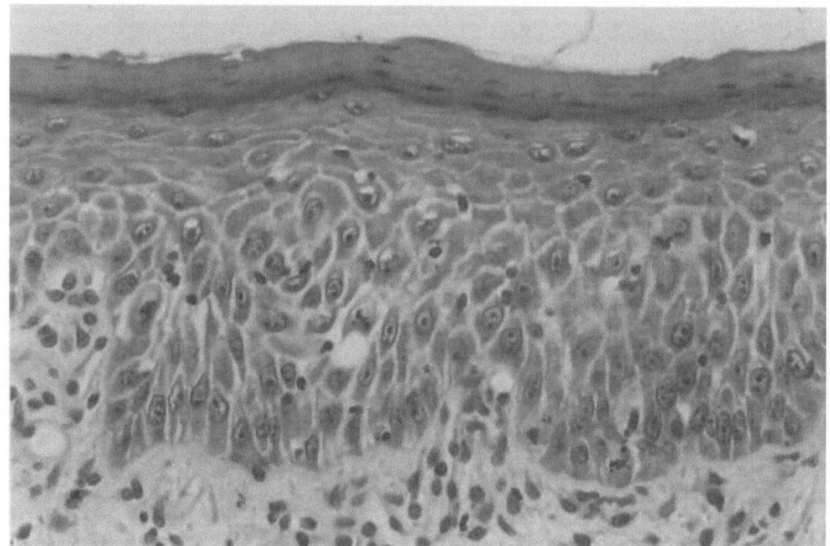

Fig. 77. *Reactive or regenerative epithelial atypia*

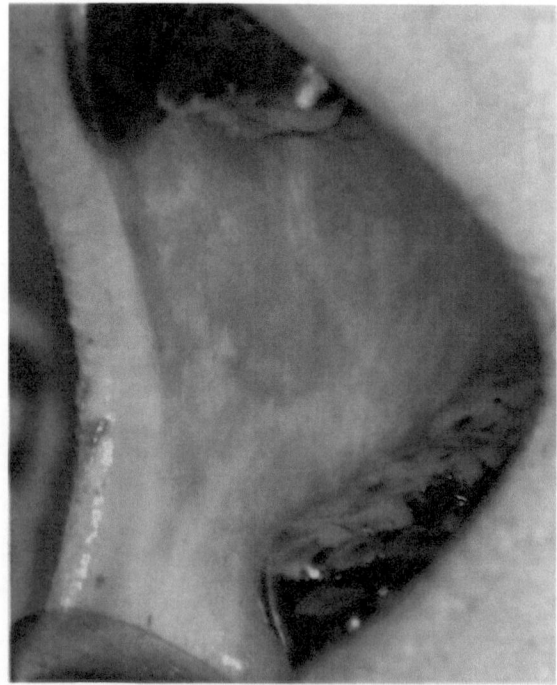

Fig. 78. *Oral submucous fibrosis.* Areas of blanching in buccal mucosa and vertical subepithelial fibrous band in commissure region

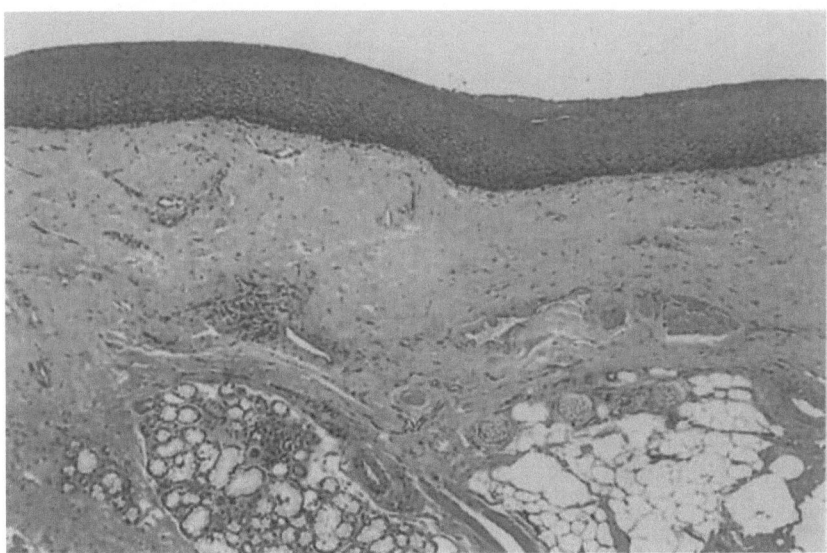

Fig. 79. *Oral submucous fibrosis.* Dense aggregation of collagen in subepithelial region extending into underlying fat

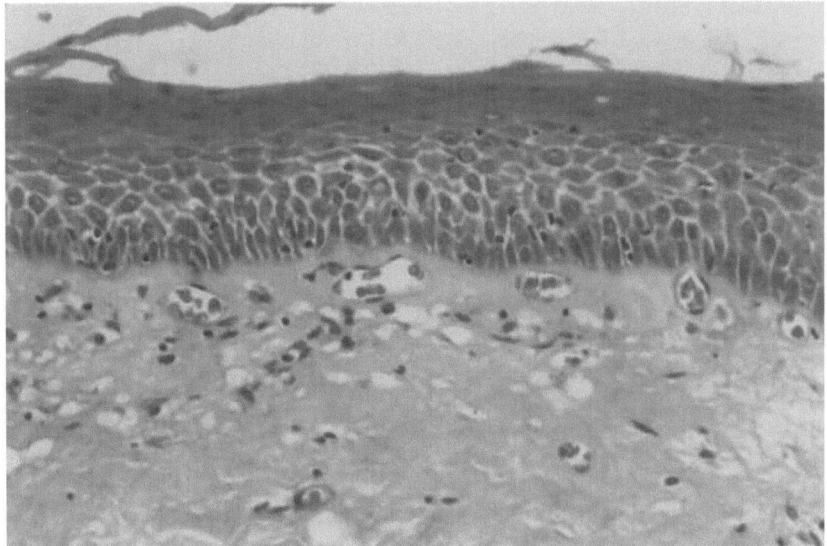

Fig. 80. *Oral submucous fibrosis.* Mild squamous epithelial dysplasia in overlying stratified squamous epithelium

Subject Index

	Pages	Figures
Actinic keratosis	27	–
Acute pseudomembranous candidiasis	27	70
Adenoid squamous cell carcinoma	15	18, 19
Adenosquamous carcinoma	16	21
Adjunctive techniques	3	–
Aetiology	3	–
Aspirin burn	27	64
Atypia, reactive and regenerative	29	77
Basaloid squamous cell carcinoma	14	16, 17
Candidiasis		
acute pseudomembranous	27	70
chronic hyperplastic	20	36–38
erythematous	28	71
Carcinoma		
adenosquamous	16	21
spindle cell	15	20
squamous cell	11	6–13
undifferentiated	16	22
verrucous	13	14, 15
Carcinoma in situ, squamous cell	26	56
Cheek biting	27	62, 63
Chievitz, juxtaoral organ of	19	35
Chronic hyperplastic candidiasis	20	36–38
Clinical presentation of oral cancer	6	1–5
Condyloma acuminatum	21	–
Discoid lupus erythematosus	17, 31	27, 28
Epidemiology	3	–
Epidermolysis bullosa	31	–
Epithelial dysplasia, squamous	25	53–55
Erosive lichen planus	28, 30	72, 73
Erythematous candidiasis	28	71
Erythroleukoplakia	23	47
Erythroplakia	24	48

	Pages	Figures
Focal epithelial hyperplasia	28	74–76
Frictional keratosis	27	59
Glossitis, median rhomboid	18	29, 30
Granular cell tumour	17	26
Hairy leukoplakia	22, 27	67–69
Histological grading	2, 11	6–9
Hyperkeratosis	24	50–52
Juxtaoral organ of Chievitz	19	35
Keratoacanthoma	18	31, 32
Keratosis		
actinic	27	–
chevron-like	25	52
frictional	27	59
hyperortho-	24	50
hyperpara-	25	51
solar	27	–
Leukoplakia	21	43–47
hairy	27	67–69
homogeneous	22	43, 44
non-homogeneous	23	45, 46
Lichen planus	27, 28, 30	65, 66, 72, 73
erosive	28, 30	72, 73
Lichenoid reaction	27	57, 58
Lupus erythematosus, discoid	17, 31	27, 28
Median rhomboid glossitis	18	29, 30
Microinvasive squamous cell carcinoma	13	11
Morsicatio buccarum	27	62, 63
Necrotizing sialometaplasia	19	33, 34
Oral cancer, clinical presentation	6	1–5
Oral submucous fibrosis	30	78–80
Palatal keratosis	24	49
Papillary hyperplasia	16	23–25
Papillary squamous cell carcinoma	13, 14	12, 13
Precancerous conditions	29	65, 66, 72, 73, 78–80

	Pages	Figures
Precancerous lesions		
clinical classification	21	43–49
histological classification	24	53–56
Proliferative verrucous leukoplakia	14, 23	–
Reactive and regenerative atypia	29	77
Red lesions resembling erythroplakia	28	71–73
Reverse smoking, palatal keratosis in	24	49
Sialometaplasia, necrotizing	19	33, 34
Sideropenic dysphagia	29	–
Solar keratosis	27	–
Spindle cell carcinoma	15	20
Squamous cell carcinoma	11	6–13
adenoid	15	18, 19
basaloid	14	16, 17
benign lesions resembling	16	23–42
microinvasive	13	11
papillary	13, 14	12, 13
Squamous cell carcinoma in situ	26	56
Squamous epithelial dysplasia	25	53–55
Submucous fibrosis, oral	30	78–80
Syphilis	30	–
Thrush	27	70
TNM classification	3, 33	–
Undifferentiated carcinoma	16	22
Verruca vulgaris	21	41, 42
Verruciform xanthoma	20	39, 40
Verrucous carcinoma	13	14, 15
Verrucous hyperplasia	14	–
White lesions resembling leukoplakia	27	57–70
White sponge naevus	27	60, 61
Xanthoma, verruciform	20	39, 40
Xeroderma pigmentosum	31	–

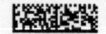